MORE 4U!

Here's what you get:

- Full text of EVERY issue from 2002 to NOW
- Figures, tables, drawings, references and more
- Searchable: find what you need fast

Search [All Clinics ▼] for [ ] [GO]

- Linked to MEDLINE and Elsevier journals
- E-alerts

INDIVIDUAL SUBSCRIBERS

LOG ON TODAY. IT'S FAST AND EASY.

Click Register and follow instructions

You'll need your account number

Your subscriber account number is on your mailing label

This is your copy of:

THE CLINICS OF NORTH AMERICA

| CXXX | 2296532-2 | 2 | Mar 05 |

J.H. DOE, MD
531 MAIN STREET
CENTER CITY, NY 10001-001

BOUGHT A SINGLE ISSUE? Sorry, you won't be able to access full text online. Please subscribe today to get complete content by contacting customer service at 800 645 2452 (US and Canada) or 407 345 4000 (outside US and Canada) or via email at elsols@elsevier.com.

NEW!

Now also available for INSTITUTIONS

ELSEVIER

Works/Integrates with MD Consult
Available in a variety of packages: Collections containing 14, 31 or 50 Clinics titles
Or Collection upgrade for existing MD Consult customers

Call today! 877-857-1047 or e-mail: mdc.groupinfo@elsevier.com

EMERGENCY MEDICINE CLINICS OF NORTH AMERICA

The ECG in Emergency Medicine

GUEST EDITORS
Richard A. Harrigan, MD,
William J. Brady, MD and
Theodore C. Chan, MD

February 2006 • Volume 24 • Number 1

SAUNDERS

An Imprint of Elsevier, Inc.
PHILADELPHIA   LONDON   TORONTO   MONTREAL   SYDNEY   TOKYO

**EMERGENCY MEDICINE CLINICS
OF NORTH AMERICA**
February 2006
Editor: Karen Sorensen

Volume 24, Number 1
ISSN 0733-8627
ISBN 1-4160-3377-7

The ideas and opinions expressed in *Emergency Medicine Clinics of North America* do not necessarily reflect those of the Publisher. The Publisher does not assume any responsibility for any injury and/or damage to persons or property arising out of or related to any use of the material contained in this periodical. The reader is advised to check the appropriate medical literature and the product information currently provided by the manufacturer of each drug to be administered to verify the dosage, the method and duration of administration, or contraindications. It is the responsibility of the treating physician or other health care professional, relying on independent experience and knowledge of the patient, to determine drug dosages and the best treatment for the patient. Mention of any product in this issue should not be construed as endorsement by the contributors, editors, or the Publisher of the product or manufacturers' claims.

Emergency Medicine Clinics of North America (ISSN 0733-8627) is published quarterly by W.B. Saunders Company. Corporate and Editorial Offices: 1600 John F. Kennedy Boulevard, Suite 1800, Philadelphia, PA 19103-2899. Accounting and Circulation Offices: 6277 Sea Harbor Drive, Orlando, FL 32887-4800. Periodicals postage paid at Orlando, FL 32862, and additional mailing offices. Subscription prices are $175.00 per year (US individuals), $275.00 per year (US institutions), $235.00 per year (international individuals), $325.00 per year (international institutions), $215.00 per year (Canadian individuals), and $325.00 per year (Canadian institutions). International air speed delivery is included in all *Clinics'* subscription prices. All prices are subject to change without notice. POSTMASTER: Send address changes to *Emergency Medicine Clinics of North America*, W.B. Saunders Company, Periodicals Fulfillment, Orlando, FL 32887-4800. **Customer Service: 1-800-654-2452 (US). From outside of the US, call 1-407-345-4000. E-mail: hhspcs@harcourt.com.**

Emergency Medicine Clinics of North America is covered in *Index Medicus, Current Contents/Clinical Medicine, EMBASE/Excerpta Medica, BIOSIS, SciSearch, CINAHL, ISI/BIOMED*, and *Research Alert.*

Printed in the United States of America.

GUEST EDITORS

RICHARD A. HARRIGAN, MD, Associate Professor, Department of Emergency Medicine, Temple University Hospital and School of Medicine, Philadelphia, Pennsylvania

WILLIAM J. BRADY, MD, Professor and Vice Chair, Department of Emergency Medicine, University of Virginia School of Medicine, Charlottesville, Virginia

THEODORE C. CHAN, MD, Professor, Clinical Medicine, Medical Director, Department of Emergency Medicine, University of California, San Diego, California

CONTRIBUTORS

WILLIAM J. BRADY, MD, Professor and Vice Chair, Department of Emergency Medicine, University of Virginia School of Medicine, Charlottesville, Virginia

TAYLOR Y. CARDALL, MD, Attending Emergency Physician, Scottsdale Emergency Associates, Scottsdale, Arizona.

THEODORE C. CHAN, MD, Professor, Clinical Medicine, Medical Director, Department of Emergency Medicine, University of California, San Diego, California

JENNIFER S. CLARK, MD, Chief Resident, Department of Emergency Medicine, Temple University School of Medicine, Philadelphia, Pennsylvania

ROBERT COWAN MD, Emergency Medicine, Virtua Memorial Hospital, Mount Holly, New Jersey

DAWN DEMANGONE, MD, Assistant Professor of Emergency Medicine, Temple University School of Medicine, Philadelphia, Pennsylvania

DAVID L. ELDRIDGE, MD, Assistant Professor, Department of Pediatrics, Brody School of Medicine, East Carolina University, Greenville, North Carolina

J. LEE GARVEY, MD, Medical Director, Chest Pain Evaluation Center, Department of Emergency Medicine, Carolinas Medical Center, Charlotte, North Carolina

RICHARD A. HARRIGAN, MD, Associate Professor, Department of Emergency Medicine, Temple University Hospital and School of Medicine, Philadelphia, Pennsylvania

CHRISTOPHER P. HOLSTEGE, MD, FACEP, FAAEM, FACMT, Director, Division of Medical Toxicology and Blue Ridge Poison Center, Associate Professor, Departments of Emergency Medicine and Pediatrics, University of Virginia, Charlottesville, Virginia

AMAL MATTU, MD, Associate Professor and Program Director, Emergency Medicine Residency, University of Maryland School of Medicine, Baltimore, Maryland

MyPHUONG MITARAI, MD, Department of Surgery/Division of Emergency Medicine, University of Maryland School of Medicine, Baltimore, Maryland

MARC L. POLLACK, MD, PhD, Research Director, Department of Emergency Medicine, York Hospital, York, Pennsylvania

SRI O. RAO, MD, Division of Pediatric Cardiology, Children's Hospital and Health Center, San Diego, California

ROBERT L. ROGERS, MD, Assistant Professor and Associate Program Director, Emergency Medicine Residency, Director of Undergraduate Medical Education, Department of Surgery/Division of Emergency Medicine and Department of Medicine; Combined Emergency Medicine/Internal Medicine Residency, University of Maryland School of Medicine, Baltimore, Maryland

ADAM K. ROWDEN, DO, Medical Toxicology Fellow, Division of Medical Toxicology and Blue Ridge Poison Center, Department of Emergency Medicine, University of Virginia, Charlottesville, Virginia

GHAZALA Q. SHARIEFF, MD, FACEP, FAAEM, FAAP, Associate Clinical Professor, Children's Hospital and Health Center/University of California–San Diego, San Diego, California; Director of Pediatric Emergency Medicine, Palomar-Pomerado Hospitals/California Emergency Physicians, San Diego, California

STEPHEN W. SMITH, MD, Faculty Emergency Physician, Department of Emergency Medicine, Hennepin County Medical Center; Associate Professor of Emergency Medicine, University of Minnesota School of Medicine, Minneapolis, Minnesota

SARAH A. STAHMER, MD, FACEP, Associate Professor, Emergency Medicine; Residency Director, Cooper Hospital/University Medical Center, Camden, New Jersey

JACOB W. UFBERG, MD, Emergency Medicine Residency Program Director, Assistant Professor of Emergency Medicine, Department of Emergency Medicine, Temple University School of Medicine, Philadelphia, Pennsylvania

DAVID A. WALD, DO, Associate Professor of Emergency Medicine; Director of Undergraduate Medical Education, Department of Emergency Medicine, Temple University School of Medicine, Philadelphia, Pennsylvania

WAYNE WHITWAM, MD, Fellow, Electrophysiology, Division of Cardiology, Department of Internal Medicine, University of California, San Diego, California

CONTENTS

> Bradydysrhythimas include sinus bradycardia, junctional brady-
> cardia, and idioventricular rhythm, which can be distinguished
> by examining the tracing for the presence or absence of P waves,
> noting the morphology of these P waves, and determining the
> width of the QRS complex. Sinoatrial blocks may occur in either
> first, second, or third degree varieties. Only second degree sinoatrial
> block can be detected on the 12-lead ECG. Sinus pause and sinus
> arrest may mimic second degree sinoatrial block, but their period-
> icity is irregular. The cyclic variability of sinus arrhythmia is
> unique; as with the other bradydysrhythmias, it may be innocent
> or pathologic depending upon clinical circumstances. Atrioventric-
> ular blocks may occur, and, similar to sinoatrial blocks, they are
> also categorized as first-, second-, or third degree. These are of
> greater clinical relevance than their sinoatrial counterparts.

> Tachydysrhythmias arise from different mechanisms that can be
> characterized as being caused by re-entrant circuits, enhanced or
> abnormal automaticity, or triggered after-depolarizations. The ap-
> proach to the tachydysrhythmia should begin with distinguishing

sinus from non-sinus rhythms, then assessing QRS complex width and regularity. This article review tachydysrhythmias.

There are multiple types of intraventricular conduction abnormalities, each with its own unique clinical significance. It is useful to categorize conduction abnormalities, or blocks, by the number of fascicles involved. This article reviews intraventricular conduction abnormalities.

Despite technologic advances in many diagnostic fields, the 12-lead ECG remains the basis for early identification and management of an acute coronary syndrome. This article reviews the use of the ECG in acute coronary syndromes.

This article reviews the ST segment and T wave abnormalities seen in non-acute coronary syndrome (ACS) electrocardiograph presentations. Particular emphasis is placed on the distinction of these non-ACS syndromes from acute coronary syndrome related ST segment and or T wave change.

The electrocardiogram reflects changes to the heart beyond those seen in acute myocardial infarction and acute coronary syndromes. Diseases of the pericardium and heart muscle such as pericarditis, myocarditis, and pericardial effusion have characteristic manifestations. Hypertensive heart disease is associated with a variety of changes on the electrocardiogram, as is valvular heart disease. Cardiac rhythm disturbances have been associated with the Brugada syndrome and the long QT syndrome, both of which have telltale findings on the electrocardiogram. The manifestations of dextrocardia, although rare, should be familiar to those who interpret electrocardiograms. Transplanted hearts also feature classic changes, both in health and in stages of rejection. The various electrocardiographic manifestations of these noncoronary heart diseases are reviewed here.

include familiarity with the age-related normal findings in heart rate, intervals, axis, and waveform morphologies; an understanding of cardiac physiologic changes associated with age and maturation, particularly the adaptation from right to left ventricular predominance; and a rudimentary understanding of common pediatric dysrhythmias and findings associated with congenital heart diseases.

The electrocardiogram (ECG) continues to be a critical component of the evaluation of patients who have signs and symptoms of emergency cardiac conditions. This tool is now approximately 100 years old and has been a standard in clinical practice for more than half a century. Application of new signal processing techniques and an expansion in the use of additional leads allows clinicians to extract more and more information from the cardiac electrical activity. An understanding of the technology inherent in the recording of ECGs allows one to more fully understand the benefits and limitation of electrocardiography.

This article includes a discussion of limb electrode misconnection, precordial electrode misconnection and misplacement, and electrocardiographic artifact.

FORTHCOMING ISSUES

RECENT ISSUES

GOAL STATEMENT

The goal of *Emergency Medicine Clinics of North America* is to keep practicing physicians up to date with current clinical practice in emergency medicine by providing timely articles reviewing the state of the art in patient care.

ACCREDITATION

The *Emergency Medical Clinics of North America* is planned and implemented in accordance with the Essential Areas and Policies of the Accreditation Council for Continuing Medical Education (ACCME) through the joint sponsorship of the University of Virginia School of Medicine and Elsevier. The University of Virginia School of Medicine is accredited by the ACCME to provide continuing medical education for physicians.

The University of Virginia School of Medicine designates this educational activity for a maximum of 60 category 1 credits per year, 15 category 1 credits per issue, toward the AMA Physician's Recognition Award. Each physician should claim only those credits that he/she actually spent in the activity.

The American Medical Association has determined that physicians not licensed in the US who participate in this CME activity are eligible for AMA PRA category 1 credit.

Category 1 credit can be earned by reading the text material, taking the CME examination online at http://www.theclinics.com/home/cme, and completing the evaluation. After taking the test, you will be required to review any and all incorrect answers. Following completion of the test and evaluation, your credit will be awarded and you may print your certificate.

FACULTY DISCLOSURE/CONFLICT OF INTEREST

The University of Virginia School of Medicine, as an ACCME accredited provider, endorses and strives to comply with the Accreditation Council for Continuing Medical Education (ACCME) Standards of Commercial Support, Commonwealth of Virginia statutes, University of Virginia policies and procedures, and associated federal and private regulations and guidelines on the need for disclosure and monitoring of proprietary and financial interests that may affect the scientific integrity and balance of content delivered in continuing medical education activities under our auspices.

The University of Virginia School of Medicine requires that all CME activities accredited through this institution be developed independently and be scientifically rigorous, balanced and objective in the presentation/discussion of its content, theories and practices.

All authors/editors participating in an accredited CME activity are expected to disclose to the readers relevant financial relationships with commercial entities occurring within the past 12 months (such as grants or research support, employee, consultant, stock holder, member of speakers bureau, etc.). The University of Virginia School of Medicine will employ appropriate mechanisms to resolve potential conflicts of interest to maintain the standards of fair and balanced education to the reader. Questions about specific strategies can be directed to the Office of Continuing Medical Education, University of Virginia School of Medicine, Charlottesville, Virginia.

The authors/editors listed below have identified no professional or financial affiliations for themselves or their spouse/partner:
Taylor Y. Cardall, MD; Theodore C. Chan, MD; Jennifer S. Clark, MD; Robert Cowan, MD; Dawn Demangone, MD; David L. Eldridge, MD; Lee Garvey, MD; Richard A. Harrigan, MD; Christopher P. Holstege, MD; Amal Mattu, MD; MyPhuong Mitarai, MD; Marc L. Pollack, MD, PhD; Sri O. Rao, MD; Richard L. Rogers, MD, FACEP, FAAEM, FACP; Adam Rowden, DO; Ghazala Q. Sharieff, MD, FACEP, FAAP, FAAEM; Stephen W. Smith, MD, FAECP; Karen Sorensen, Acquisitions Editor; Sarah A. Stahmer, MD; Jacob W. Ufberg, MD; David A. Wald, DO; and Wayne Whitwam, MD, ABIM.

The author listed below has identified the following professional or financial affiliation for himself or spouse/partner:
William J. Brady, MD is Medical Director and owner of ECG Consultants, Inc., an educational company that is in the design phase.

Disclosure of Discussion of non-FDA approved uses for pharmaceutical products and/or medical devices:
The University of Virginia School of Medicine, as an ACCME provider, requires that all faculty presenters identify and disclose any "off label" uses for pharmaceutical and medical device products. The University of Virginia School of Medicine recommends that each physician fully review all the available data on new products or procedures prior to instituting them with patients.

TO ENROLL

To enroll in the Emergency Medicine Clinics of North America Continuing Medical Education program, call customer service at 1-800-654-2452 or visit us online at www.theclinics.com/home/cme. The CME program is available to subscribers for an additional fee of $195.00

EMERGENCY
MEDICINE
CLINICS OF
NORTH AMERICA

ELSEVIER
SAUNDERS

Emerg Med Clin N Am 24 (2006) xi–xii

Preface

The ECG in Emergency Medicine

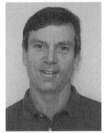 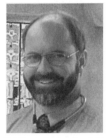 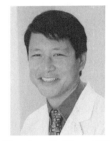

Richard A. Harrigan, MD   William J. Brady, MD   Theodore C. Chan, MD
Guest Editors

The electrocardiogram (ECG) is an ideal tool for the practice of emergency medicine—it is non-invasive, inexpensive, easy to use, and it yields a wealth of information. All emergency physicians interpret multiple ECGs every day–and at times the most critical decisions of any given day are based on ECG interpretation at the bedside, such as in the assessment of the patients with chest pain, dyspnea, or even shock. However, although the "high profile" disease states—such as acute coronary syndrome—classically are linked with this indispensable tool, we use the ECG for much more.

Although traditionally the ECG is thought of as a cardiologist's tool, it is really the domain of any medical practitioner making real-time assessments of patients—the emergency physician, the internist, the family practitioner, the intensivist, to name a few. As such, we all must become very comfortable with the many facets and subtleties of ECG interpretation. We should be expert in the urgent and emergent interpretation of the ECG. It is our hope that this issue of the *Emergency Medicine Clinics of North America* will help the physician on the front lines of patient care understand the complex wealth of information delivered by this relatively simple test.

In this issue, we examine the ECG in traditional and nontraditional realms. Diagnosis of dysrhythmia and acute coronary syndromes is an obvious focus of this text. Several articles take an in-depth look at other morphologic issues we are often confronted with on the ECG; namely intraventricular conduction delays, the manifestations of electronic cardiac pacemakers, and the subtleties of ST segment/T wave changes as they pertain to the many syndromes that cause them. The issue also includes several

doi:10.1016/j.emc.2005.08.002   *emed.theclinics.com*

articles on electrocardiographic manifestations of noncoronary disease, both cardiac and systemic. The ECG is also examined in subpopulations important to the emergency medicine practitioner: the child and the poisoned patient. Finally, more atypical topics of ECG interpretation are included; we offer an article on the detection of electrode misconnection and artifact, and look toward the horizon with a consideration of newer techniques and technologies.

While working on this issue of the *Emergency Medicine Clinics of North America,* we considered not only healthcare provider education, but the constraints of rendering patient care in the emergency setting. We would like to recognize all emergency health care providers for their dedicated work for individuals in need. This work is performed at times under extreme circumstances with minimal information and resource. And yet, the outcome is most often positive. We should indeed all be proud of our profession.

We are happy to present a broad range of talented authors from across the country, and we feel they have provided you with an excellent, in-depth discussion of the ECG. It is our hope that you will enjoy this issue on *The ECG in Emergency Medicine*, and that it will serve as informative reading to you as well as a valued reference for the future.

Richard A. Harrigan, MD
Department of Emergency Medicine
Temple University Hospital and School of Medicine
Jones 1005 Park Avenue and Ontario Street
Philadelphia, PA 19140

E-mail address: richard.harrigan@tuhs.temple.edu

William J. Brady, MD
University of Virginia School of Medicine
Department of Emergency Medicine
PO Box 800309
Charlottesville, VA 22908

E-mail address: Wb4z@virginia.edu

Theodore C. Chan, MD
UCSD
Department of Emergency Medicine
200 West Harbor Drive, #8676
San Diego, CA 92103

E-mail address: tcchan@ucsd.edu

ELSEVIER
SAUNDERS

Emerg Med Clin N Am 24 (2006) xiii

EMERGENCY
MEDICINE
CLINICS OF
NORTH AMERICA

Dedication

The ECG in Emergency Medicine

With love and thanks to my sister, Joan, who is and always has been there—ahead of me in many ways, beside me and behind me in so many others.

Richard A. Harrigan, MD

I'd like to thank my wife, King, and children, Lauren, Anne, Chip, and Katherine, for being wonderful, supportive, and understanding—you guys are my inspiration! My parents, JoAnn and Bill Brady, must also be included in this list.

The Emergency Medicine residents and Medical Students at the University of Virginia are awesome and deserving of my thanks, both for their incredibly hard work with our patients and for providing the impetus to explore the ECG.

I must also thank Dr. Marcus Martin for his support, guidance, and extreme patience—it's appreciated more than I can say.

William J. Brady, MD

To Diana for her love and support, and my wonderful children, Taylor, James and Lauren

Theodore C. Chan, MD

Richard A. Harrigan, MD
William J. Brady, MD
Theodore C. Chan, MD
Guest Editors

doi:10.1016/j.emc.2005.08.001   *emed.theclinics.com*

EMERGENCY
MEDICINE
CLINICS OF
NORTH AMERICA

ELSEVIER
SAUNDERS

Emerg Med Clin N Am 24 (2006) 1–9

Bradydysrhythmias and Atrioventricular Conduction Blocks

Jacob W. Ufberg, MD*, Jennifer S. Clark, MD

*Department of Emergency Medicine, Temple University School of Medicine, 10th Floor,
Jones Hall, 3401 North Broad Street, Philadelphia, PA 19140, USA*

Bradydysrhythmias

Bradycardia is defined as a ventricular rate less than 60 beats per minute (bpm). Sinus bradycardia exists when a P wave precedes each QRS complex. This QRS complex is usually narrow (less than 0.120 seconds) because the impulse originates from a supraventricular focus (Fig. 1). On ECG, the P-P interval in sinus bradycardia closely matches the R-R interval, because the P wave is always preceding a QRS complex and the rate is regular. Each P wave within a given lead has the same morphology and axis, because the same atrial focus is generating the P wave.

There are specific incidences in which, despite the supraventricular focus, the QRS is widened (greater than 0.12 seconds). An example of this is a bundle branch block (right or left) in which the QRS complex is wide, but each QRS complex is still preceded by a P wave, and thus the underlying rhythm is still considered sinus bradycardia. Clues to differentiate this on ECG are that the PR interval usually remains constant and the QRS morphology is typical of a bundle branch block pattern.

Other ECG rhythms may seem like sinus bradycardia but in fact do not meet the definition as mentioned (see section on sinoatrial block).

Junctional rhythm is another example of a supraventricular rhythm in which the QRS complex morphology is usually narrow (less than 0.12 seconds) and regular. This is distinguished from sinus bradycardia on ECG because it is not associated with preceding P waves or any preceding atrial aberrant rhythms. On ECG, a junctional escape rate is usually 40–60 bpm, because the impulse is generated below the SA node, at the atrioventricular (AV) junction. A junctional rhythm with a rate slower than 40 bpm is termed

---

* Corresponding author.
E-mail address: ufbergjw@tuhs.temple.edu (J.W. Ufberg).

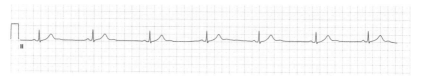

Fig. 1. Sinus bradycardia. The rate is 40 bpm. There are P waves preceding each QRS complex, and the QRS duration is less than 0.12 seconds.

junctional bradycardia, and a junctional rhythm with a rate faster than 60 bpm is termed an accelerated junctional rhythm or a junctional tachycardia; this reflects usurpation of pacemaker control from the sinus node (Fig. 2).

There are times when there are P waves evident on the ECG of patients who have a junctional rhythm, but unlike normal sinus rhythm or sinus bradycardia, these P waves are not conducted in an anterograde fashion. These are termed P′ waves and may appear before, during (in which case they are obscured), or after the QRS complex, depending on when the atrium is captured by the impulse emanating from the AV junction. Retrograde atrial capture is affected by the origin of the AV junctional impulse (physical location of the pacemaker, whether it is high, middle, or lower AV node) and the speed of conduction. As in sinus bradycardia, there are also times in which the QRS morphology is widened (greater than 0.12 seconds) because of a right or left bundle branch block.

Idioventricular rhythms are regular, but unlike sinus bradycardia or junctional rhythms, they are always characterized by a wide QRS complex (greater than 0.12 seconds), because their origin lies somewhere within the

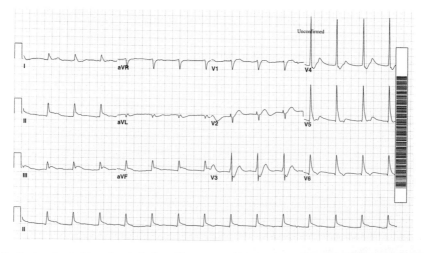

Fig. 2. Accelerated junctional rhythm. There are no P waves preceding each QRS complex. The QRS complex is narrow. This tracing is from a patient suffering from an acute inferior wall myocardial infarction; note the ST segment elevation in leads II, III, and aVF.

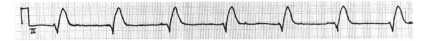

Fig. 3. Idioventricular rhythm. The rate is 40 bpm with a widened QRS complex (130 ms). There is no evidence of P waves on this rhythm strip.

ventricles (Fig. 3). On ECG, the rate is usually 20–40 bpm except for accelerated idioventricular rhythms (rate greater than 40 bpm).

Sinoatrial (SA) blocks result when there is an abnormality between the conduction of the impulse from the heart's normal pacemaker (SA node) to the surrounding atrium. Because there is a wide range of severity of dysfunction, there are many ECG findings associated with SA blocks (also called SA exit blocks) (Fig. 4) [1]. As with AV block, SA block is characterized as first-, second-, and third-degree, with second-degree blocks subclassified as type I and type II.

First-degree SA block represents an increased time for the SA node's impulse to reach and depolarize the rest of the atrium (ie, form a P wave). Because impulse origination from the SA node does not produce a deflection on the 12-lead ECG, there are no abnormalities seen on the 12-lead tracing with first-degree SA block.

Second-degree SA block is evident on the surface ECG. Second-degree SA block type I occurs when there is a progressively increasing interval for each SA nodal impulse to depolarize the atrial myocardium (ie, cause a P wave), which continues to lengthen until the SA node's impulse does not depolarize the atrium at all. This is manifested by gradual shortening of the P-P interval with an eventual "dropped" P-QRS-T complex. It can be recognized by "grouped beatings" of the P-QRS-T complexes, or may manifest as irregular sinus rhythm (a sinus rhythm with pauses) on the ECG.

Second-degree SA block type II occurs when there is a consistent interval between the SA node impulse and the depolarization of the atrium with an occasional SA nodal impulse that is not conducted at all. On the ECG, there is a dropped P-QRS-T complex with a P-P interval surrounding the pause that is two to four times the length of the baseline P-P interval [2].

Second-degree SA block with 2:1 conduction is seen on ECG when every other impulse from the SA node causes atrial depolarization while the other is dropped. The ECG findings associated with this block are difficult. It is impossible to differentiate this from sinus bradycardia unless the beginning or termination of the SA block is caught on ECG. This manifests on ECG as a distinct halving (beginning) or doubling (termination) of the baseline rate.

Third-degree SA block occurs when none of the SA nodal impulses depolarize the atrium. This appears as a junctional rhythm with no P waves on the 12 lead tracing, because the focus now responsible for depolarization of the ventricles lies below the SA node. Sometimes there is a long pause on the ECG until a normal sinus rhythm is resumed. This pause is difficult

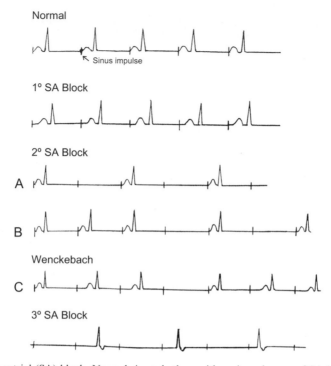

Fig. 4. Sinoatrial (SA) block. Normal sinus rhythms with various degrees of SA block. Sinus impulses not seen on the body surface ECG are represented by the vertical lines. With first-degree SA block, although there is prolongation of the interval between the sinus impulses and the P wave, such a delay cannot be detected on the ECG. (*A*) Persistent 2:1 SA block cannot be distinguished from marked sinus bradycardia. (*B*) The diagnosis of second-degree SA block depends on the presence of pause or pauses that are the multiple of the basic P-P interval. (*C*) When there is a Wenckebach phenomenon, there is gradual shortening of the P-P interval before the pause. With third-degree SA block, the ECG records only the escape rhythm. *Used with permission from* Suawicz B, Knilans TK. Chou's electrocardiography in clinical practice. 5th edition. Philadelphia: WB Saunders; 2001. p. 321.

to distinguish from sinus pause or arrest. All pauses in SA blocks, however, should be a multiple (two to four times the length) of the P-P intervals on the ECG (see section on sinus pause/arrest for more details).

Sinus pause and sinus arrest are characterized by the failure of the SA node to form an impulse. Although sinus pause refers to a brief failure and a sinus arrest refers to a more prolonged failure of the SA node, there are no universally accepted definitions to differentiate the two. Because of this, they are often used interchangeably to describe the same cardiac event (Fig. 5) [3].

On ECG there is an absence of the P-QRS-T complex, resulting in a pause of undetermined length. Sinus pause may be preceded by any of these rhythms, the origin of which is in the atrium: sinus beats, ectopic atrial beats, and ectopic atrial tachycardia. Or it may appear on the ECG with

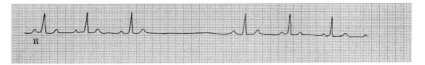

Fig. 5. Sinus pause. This rhythm strip demonstrates P waves preceding each QRS complex until a P-QRS-T complex is dropped. Notice the underlying rhythm is sinus bradycardia before and after the sinus pause. The P-P interval during the sinus pause is not a multiple of the baseline P-P interval on the ECG, which helps differentiate this rhythm from a second-degree SA block.

a junctional escape rhythm in which an AV nodal impulse has suppressed the sinus node [4]. After the sinus pause/arrest is seen on the ECG, the rhythm that follows also varies greatly. The sinus node most often resumes pacemaker activity and a normal sinus rhythm is seen. In cases in which it fails, however, the escape rhythm seen is usually from the AV node. If the AV node fails, the next pacemaker to take would result in an idioventricular rhythm. If all of these fail to generate an escape rhythm, the result is asystole.

The difficulty remains in distinguishing sinus pause/arrest from SA block. The biggest apparent difference between the two rhythms is the P-P interval. During sinus pause, the P-P interval is not a multiple of the baseline P-P interval. In SA block, however, the P-P interval should be a multiple of the baseline P-P interval.

Sinus arrhythmia is seen electrocardiographically as a gradual, cyclical variation in the P-P interval (Fig. 6). The longest P-P interval exceeds the shortest P-P interval by more than 0.16 seconds. Most commonly this occurs as a normal variation caused by respiratory variability; the sinus rate increases with inspiration and decreases during expiration [5]. In elderly individuals, it may be a manifestation of sick sinus syndrome.

Sick sinus syndrome is a collective term that includes a range of SA node dysfunction that manifests in various different ways on the ECG, including inappropriate sinus bradycardia, sinus arrhythmia, sinus pause/arrest, SA exit block, AV junctional (escape) rhythm (all discussed earlier), and the bradycardia-tachycardia syndrome. Bradycardia-tachycardia syndrome (or tachy-brady syndrome) is defined by bradycardic rhythms alternating with episodes of tachycardia. These tachycardic rhythms usually are supraventricular in origin but at times may be accelerated junctional or ventricular rhythms. A distinguishing finding of this syndrome on ECG, though difficult to capture, is the transition from the termination of the tachydysrhythmia

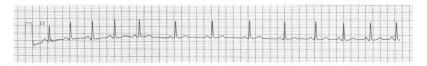

Fig. 6. Sinus arrhythmia. Here demonstrated in an elderly patient, this sinus arrhythmia most likely is caused by sick sinus syndrome.

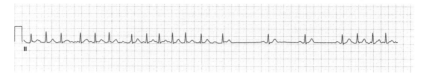

Fig. 7. Tachycardia-bradycardia syndrome. This ECG from a woman with sick sinus syndrome demonstrates initial atrial fibrillation with a rapid ventricular response that alternates with sinus bradycardia.

back to a sinus nodal rhythm. Often, severe sinus bradycardia, sinus pause/ arrest, SA block, or junctional rhythm occur first until the sinus mechanism recovers (Fig. 7).

Atrioventricular block

Like SA block, AV block can be partial or complete and also is divided into first-, second-, and third-degree varieties. Second-degree, again similar to SA block, is divided into Mobitz type I (Wenckebach AV block) and Mobitz type II. A clue to differentiating between SA blocks and AV blocks is remembering where the conduction delay is occurring. In SA block, the dysfunction occurs between the SA node and the atrial myocardium; thus, there is a dropped P-QRS-T complex. In AV block, conduction is altered between the atrium and the ventricle, causing a prolonged PR interval and a dropped QRS-T complex (eventually a P wave occurs without a QRS-T behind it).

First-degree AV block is defined as a prolonged PR interval (greater than 0.20 seconds) that remains constant. The P wave and QRS complex have normal morphology, and a P wave precedes each QRS complex (Fig. 8). The lengthening of the PR interval results from a conduction delay from within the atrium, the AV node, or the His-Purkinje system. Most patients have a narrow QRS complex (less than 0.12 seconds), which indicates a block in the AV node, but occasionally there is a widened QRS complex associated with a delay in lower cardiac conduction. And as with SA blocks, patients may have a wide QRS complex caused by a coexisting bundle branch block.

Second-degree AV block, Mobitz type I is characterized by normal P wave and QRS complex morphology beginning with a PR interval that

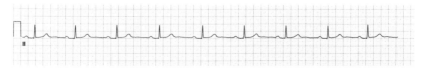

Fig. 8. First-degree AV block. This rhythm strip demonstrates sinus bradycardia. The rate is 54 bpm with every P wave followed by a QRS complex. The PR interval is constant and prolonged (0.23 seconds) with normal QRS and P wave morphology, thus meeting the definition of first-degree AV block.

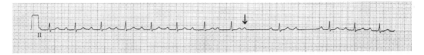

Fig. 9. Second-degree AV block, Mobitz type I. Note the PR intervals that lengthen gradually until a QRS complex is dropped ([*arrow*] denotes P wave without QRS complex to follow). Because the QRS complex is narrow, the conduction delay occurs before or within the AV node.

lengthens progressively with each cycle until an impulse does not reach the ventricles and a QRS complex is dropped (Fig. 9). This block is usually at or above the AV node. On ECG, the PR interval lengthens as the R-R interval shortens. The R-R interval that contains the dropped beat is less than two of the shortest R-R intervals seen on the ECG. Also, on the ECG rhythm strip, a grouping of beats typically is seen, especially with tachycardia; this is referred to as "grouped beating of Wenckebach" [1,6]. All four of these ECG findings are typical of Mobitz type I block but unfortunately have been observed in less than 50% of all cases reported [1,7]. What has been reported are variations on all of the above, from PR intervals not lengthening progressively to conducting all atrial impulses to the ventricles [6,7]. These variations on second-degree Mobitz type I AV block seen on ECG do not change the clinical importance of this AV block [8].

Second-degree AV block, Mobitz type II is defined by constant PR intervals that may be normal or prolonged (>0.20 seconds). Unlike Mobitz type I second-degree AV block, however, Mobitz type II blocks do not demonstrate progressive lengthening of the PR interval on the ECG before a QRS complex is dropped. Also, unlike type I second-degree AV block, the QRS complex usually is widened, because the location of this block is often infranodal. The QRS complex may be narrow, however, indicating a more proximal location of block, usually in the AV node. The magnitude of the AV block can be expressed as a ratio of P waves to QRS complexes. For example, if there are four P waves to every three QRS complexes, it would be a 4:3 block (Fig. 10) [9].

Because Mobitz type II second-degree AV block does not have progressively lengthening PR intervals, differentiating type I from type II on ECG is simple, except in the case of 2:1 block. In second-degree AV block with 2:1

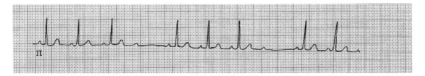

Fig. 10. Second-degree AV block, Mobitz type II. There are constant PR intervals preceding each QRS complex until a QRS complex is dropped in this rhythm strip. There are four P waves to every three QRS complexes, thus a 4:3 block.

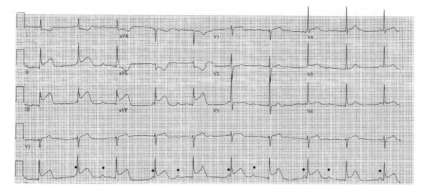

Fig. 11. Third-degree AV block. Complete heart block is seen here with P waves (*dots*) that "march" through the QRS-T complexes; at times the P waves are obscured by these other waveforms. The atrial rate (approximately 90 bpm) is faster than the escape ventricular rate (approximately 60 bpm), which is driven by the junctional pacemaker; rephrased, the P-P interval is shorter than the R-R interval, as it should be in complete heart block. Note this patient is having an acute inferior myocardial infarction, with ST segment elevation (leads II, III, and aVF) and reciprocal ST segment depression (leads aVL and I). The right coronary artery is the culprit vessel.

block, every other QRS-T is dropped (ie, two P waves for each QRS complex), so there is no opportunity to determine if the PR interval lengthens before the dropped QRS complex. If the ventricular beat is represented by a widened QRS complex, this suggests a more concerning Mobitz type II block, but ultimately it may be impossible to differentiate between the two. In that case, the physician should presume it is Mobitz type II, because it is more likely to progress to third-degree (complete) heart block.

High-grade or advanced AV block is a more clinically concerning variant of Mobitz type II block and is manifested by two or more P waves that are

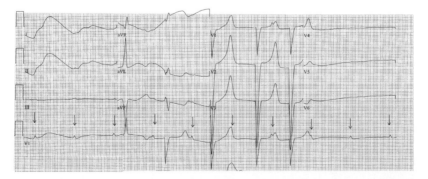

Fig. 12. Complete heart block with periods of asystole. Note that several P waves occur at first without associated QRS complexes, before an idioventricular escape rhythm ensues. P waves are denoted by *arrows*. This patient survived and received an electronic pacemaker.

not conducted. This most often implies advanced conduction disease seen in anterior infarction and has high risk for progression to complete heart block [9]. On the ECG there are usually widened QRS complexes with ventricular rates between 20 and 40 bpm.

Third-degree AV block (complete heart block) occurs when no impulses from the atria reach the ventricles. The atria and ventricles thus are functioning independently (ie, there is AV dissociation), and the atrial rate is faster than the ventricular rate because the latter is an escape rhythm (Fig. 11). The escape rhythm controlling the ventricles is usually regular because of the increased autonomic control of the ventricle compared with the sinus node [10]. The atrial impulses (P waves) "march" out on the ECG, as do the ventricular depolarizations (QRS complexes), yet they are unrelated. The ventricular rate is usually 40–60 bpm with a narrow QRS complex when it is driven by a junctional pacemaker (within the AV node). If an infra-Hisian ventricular pacemaker takes over, the QRS complexes are wide and the rate is less than 40 bpm. Ventricular escape rhythms usually are associated with a poorer prognosis and are caused more commonly by acquired (noncongenital) conditions [6]. It is also possible that no escape rhythm is generated, resulting in asystolic arrest (Fig. 12).

References

[1] Olgin JE, Zipes DP. Specific arrhythmias: diagnosis and treatment. In: Braunwald E, Zipes DP, Libby P, editors. Braunwald: heart disease: a textbook of cardiovascular medicine. 6th edition. Philadelphia: WB Saunders; 2001. p. 815–89.

[2] Sandoe E, Sigurd B. Arrhythmia—a guide to clinical electrocardiology. Verlags GmbH: Bingen Publishing Partners; 1991. p. 278–90.

[3] Shaw DB, Southall DP. Sinus node arrest and sino-atrial block. Eur Heart J 1984;5(Suppl A):83–7.

[4] Chung EK. Principles of cardiac arrhythmias. 3rd edition. Baltimore: Williams and Wilkins; 1983. p. 72–4.

[5] Applegate TE. Atrial arrhythmias. Prim Care 2000;27:677–708.

[6] Rardon DP, Miles WM, Zipes DP. Atrioventricular block and dissociation. In: Zipes DP, Jalife J, editors. Cardiac electrophysiology: from cell to bedside. 3rd edition. Philadelphia: WB Saunders; 2000. p. 451–9.

[7] Denes P, Levy L, Pick A, et al. The incidence of typical and atypical A-V Wenckebach periodicity. Am Heart J 1975;89:26–31.

[8] Hayden GE, Brady WJ, Pollack M, et al. Electrocardiographic manifestations: diagnosis of atrioventricular block in the emergency department. J Emerg Med 2004;26:95–106.

[9] Brady WJ, Harrigan RA. Diagnosis and management of bradycardia and atrioventricular block associated with acute coronary ischemia. Emerg Med Clin North Am 2001;19:371–83.

[10] Wagner GS. Intraventricular conduction abnormalities. In: Marriott's practical electrocardiography. 10th edition. Philadelphia: Lippincott Williams & Wilkins; 2001. p. 95–122.

ELSEVIER
SAUNDERS

Emerg Med Clin N Am 24 (2006) 11–40

EMERGENCY
MEDICINE
CLINICS OF
NORTH AMERICA

Tachydysrhythmias

Sarah A. Stahmer, MD*, Robert Cowan, MD

*Emergency Medicine, Cooper Hospital/University Medical Center,
One Cooper Plaza, Room 114, Camden, NJ 08103, USA*

Mechanisms of tachydysrhythmia

Correct interpretation of the electrocardiogram (ECG) is pivotal to diagnosis and management of tachydysrhythmias, because treatment options are often specific for a given dysrhythmia. Although one would like to be able to simplify the classification of tachydysrhythmias into supraventricular tachycardia (SVT) or ventricular tachycardia (VT), the growing number of treatment options and potential for adverse outcomes associated with incorrect interpretation forces one to further refine the diagnosis. It would also be immensely convenient if every dysrhythmia had a classic ECG appearance and every patient with a given dysrhythmia manifested a similar clinical presentation. Unfortunately there is wide variation in ECG appearance and clinical presentation of any dysrhythmia because of variability in the origin of the rhythm, underlying cardiac anatomy, and pre-existing ECG abnormalities. For this reason, this article not only focuses on the classic presentations of each dysrhythmia but also provides insight into the pathophysiology of the rhythm and anticipated response to maneuvers that verify or refute the working diagnosis.

The basic mechanisms of all tachydysrhythmias fall into one of three categories: re-entrant dysrhythmias, abnormal automaticity, and triggered dysrhythmias. Re-entry is the most commonly encountered mechanism of dysrhythmia. Re-entry, although typically associated with dysrhythmias arising from the atrioventricular node (AVN) and perinodal tissues, can occur essentially in any part of the heart. The primary requirement of a re-entrant circuit is the presence of two functional or anatomic pathways that differ in their speed of conduction and recovery (Fig. 1). They usually are triggered by an early beat, such as a premature atrial contraction (PAC), which finds one pathway blocked because of slow recovery and is conducted

---

* Corresponding author.
E-mail address: stahmer-sarah@cooperhealth.edu (S.A. Stahmer).

doi:10.1016/j.emc.2005.08.007   *emed.theclinics.com*

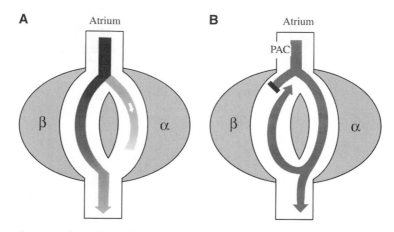

Fig. 1. Re-entry circuit. These figures depict a re-entrant circuit in the AVN with two tracts. The beta tract is the fast-conducting, slow-recovery tract that typifies normal conduction through the AVN. The alpha tract is the slow-conducting but fast-recovery pathway. (*A*) Normal conduction in which conduction comes from the atrium and splits into the two tracts. Because the beta tract is faster, it carries the signal to the ventricle before the alpha tract. (*B*) A re-entrant circuit precipitated by a PAC. The PAC finds the beta tract refractory from the prior beat (represented by the black rectangle). The signal therefore conducts down the alpha tract. Because the alpha is slower, by the time it reaches the ventricle the beta tract is no longer refractory and the signal is conducted antegrade to the ventricle and retrograde up the beta tract. On reaching the atrial end, the alpha tract (because of its fast recovery) is ready to conduct. The signal goes down the alpha tract again and the loop is completed.

down the alternate pathway, which has a faster recovery period. The wave of conduction finds the other pathway, now no longer refractory, able to conduct the beat in a retrograde fashion, and the re-entrant circuit now is established. Examples of re-entrant rhythms include AVN re-entry, orthodromic re-entrant tachycardia (ORT), and VT. The clinical response of these dysrhythmias to pharmacologic and electrical interventions depends on the characteristics of the tissue comprising the re-entrant circuit. For example, rhythms that incorporate the AVN into the re-entrant circuit are sensitive to vagal maneuvers and adenosine, whereas ventricular re-entrant tachycardias are not. The goal of therapy is to disrupt the re-entrant circuit, which can be accomplished through medications that block conduction in one limb of the circuit. There is wide variation in the responsiveness of various cardiac tissue and conduction pathways to cardiac medications, and some knowledge of the location of the pathway is important.

Dysrhythmias caused by automaticity can be particularly frustrating in that they are often incessant and do not respond predictably to electrical or pharmacologic interventions. They are caused by enhanced automaticity in fibers that have pacemaker capability or by abnormal automaticity in diseased tissue, which may arise from any portion of the heart. Enhanced normal automaticity is caused by steepening of phase 4 depolarization, resulting in premature attainment of the threshold membrane potential (Fig. 2).

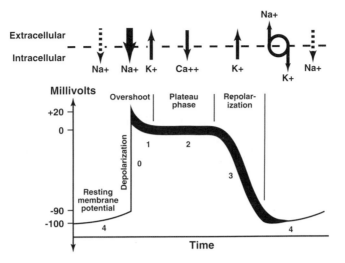

Fig. 2. Action potential duration. This is a diagram of a typical action potential for a cardiac cell that displays automaticity. At the far left the resting potential is approximately −90 to −100 mV set up by the sodium/potassium pump (*circle with arrows to the right*). Because there is slow leak of sodium (phase 4; *dashed arrows*), the cell eventually reaches the threshold. Fast sodium channels (phase 0) open, allowing sodium to enter the cell and cause depolarization. During the overshoot, potassium leaves the cell and during the plateau phase calcium ions flow into the cell. While potassium leaves the cell through potassium channels (phase 3), calcium channels close, leading to repolarization and restoration of the resting membrane potential. It is the steepness of phase 4 depolarization that determines the rate of firing of cardiac cells that act as pacemakers.

Rhythms associated with this mechanism are atrial and junctional tachycardias and often are caused by adrenergic stimulation. These rhythms are likely to respond to overdrive pacing. Abnormal automaticity is spontaneous phase 4 depolarization in tissues that normally do not demonstrate automaticity. These usually are seen in patients who have myocardial ischemia or recent cardiac surgery. Rhythms associated with this mechanism include postmyocardial infarction (MI) VT, accelerated idioventricular rhythms, and some atrial and junctional tachycardias. In general, these cannot be terminated with overdrive pacing or electrical cardioversion and frequently are resistant to pharmacologic therapy.

Triggered dysrhythmias are caused by after-depolarizations that are referred to as early and late, depending on when they arise in the action potential. They are not automatic because of their dependency on a preceding action potential. Early after-depolarizations occur during phase 3 of repolarization (Fig. 2). Conditions resulting in prolongation of the QT interval increase the risk for triggering a dysrhythmia. These dysrhythmias tend to occur in salvos and are more likely to occur when the sinus rate is slow. A classic example is torsades de pointes. Delayed after-depolarizations are caused by any condition that results in accumulation of intracellular calcium that stimulates sodium–calcium exchange. The transient influx of sodium results in oscillations of the membrane potential following completion of phase 3 repolarization. Tachydysrhythmias associated with digoxin toxicity are caused by this mechanism.

Approach to ECG interpretation of tachydysrhythmias

Differentiation among the various dysrhythmias requires an approach that is based on an understanding of basic cardiac pathophysiology. The first step is to decide whether the rhythm is a sinus tachycardia. This is usually a compensatory rhythm and the work-up should focus on identification of the precipitating condition rather than on treating the rhythm itself. For this one has to look at the patient and often a longer rhythm strip. Sinus tachycardia usually is seen in the context of a patient who is ill or in distress, reflecting inadequate cardiac stroke volume or the presence of a hyperadrenergic state from pain, fear, anxiety, or exogenous catecholamines. Another clue to the presence of a sinus tachycardia is that sinus tachycardia has no fixed rate and shows gradual variation in rate over time and in response to therapy.

A very rapid heart beat in a patient who has no other apparent problem would lead one to suspect a non-sinus rhythm. Regular dysrhythmias have a fixed unchanging rate despite changes in levels of pain and distress, whereas irregular tachydysrhythmias (such as atrial fibrillation) demonstrate beat-to-beat variability not seen in sinus tachycardia (Fig. 3).

The next decision is whether the QRS complexes are narrow or wide, with wide being defined as greater than 0.12 seconds. A narrow QRS complex indicates that there is a normal pattern of ventricular activation and the beat must originate at or above the level of the AVN. These rhythms are referred to loosely as SVTs. The presence of a wide QRS complex usually is first interpreted as a sign that the rhythm originates from the ventricle, as in VT. Alternatively, the rhythm may be supraventricular and the QRS complex is wide because of a pre-existing bundle branch block (BBB), rate-related

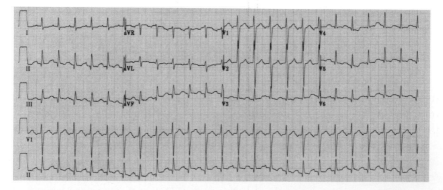

Fig. 3. Sinus tachycardia. This is a regular narrow complex tachycardia with a P wave before every QRS complex with a fixed PR interval. Telemetry reveals gradual rate changes in response to clinical condition or therapeutic interventions.

conduction aberrancy, or a ventricular-paced rhythm. Finally, conduction down a bypass tract can result in a wide QRS complex. The differential of a wide complex tachycardia is discussed later in this article. Most SVTs are narrow.

The next step in interpretation is to determine regularity. Irregular tachydysrhythmias are nearly always supraventricular in origin because of the presence of multiple atrial pacemakers or variable AV block. Irregular supraventricular dysrhythmias are sinus tachycardia with frequent PACs, atrial fibrillation, atrial flutter with variable AVN block, and multifocal atrial tachycardia.

Regular SVTs include sinus tachycardia, atrial flutter with fixed AVN block, non-sinus atrial tachycardias, re-entrant tachycardias, and junctional tachycardias. Infranodal rhythms are nearly always caused by enhanced automaticity or re-entry and usually are regular. VT is the prime example, and it is usually regular.

Regular supraventricular tachydysrhythmias

Sinus tachycardia

The ECG demonstrates a uniform P wave morphology that is upright in leads I, II, and aVF. There is a P wave before every QRS complex, with constant PR intervals. The rate is not fixed and demonstrates gradual variations in the rate in response to the etiology and interventions (Fig. 3). Rhythms commonly misinterpreted as sinus tachycardia are atrial tachycardia and atrial flutter with 2:1 AVN block. Atrial tachycardia can be distinguished from sinus tachycardia by the P waves, which often have an abnormal axis and generally do not respond to vagal maneuvers (Fig. 4). Atrial flutter with 2:1 block has a fixed rate, usually approximately 150 bpm. Vagal maneuvers may result in increased AV block and may unmask the characteristic flutter waves.

Atrial tachycardia

Atrial tachycardia is the least common and often most challenging of the regular SVTs [1–5]. It can result from various mechanisms, and the 12-lead ECG rarely provides clues to the cause. In the setting of a normal atrial myocardial tissue, the more likely mechanism is one of automaticity. Usually seen in the setting of a catecholamine surge, a single focus in the atrium has enhanced automaticity and takes over pacing from the sinoatrial (SA) node. This type of rhythm tends to accelerate to its maximal rate and is not initiated by a PAC. It typically demonstrates beat-to-beat variability during its warm-up period and decelerates gradually [1–5]. In patients who have diseased atrial tissue or who have undergone atrial surgeries, atrial tachycardia more commonly is secondary to re-entrant loops. Surgery to correct defects such as transposition of the great vessels, atrial septal defects,

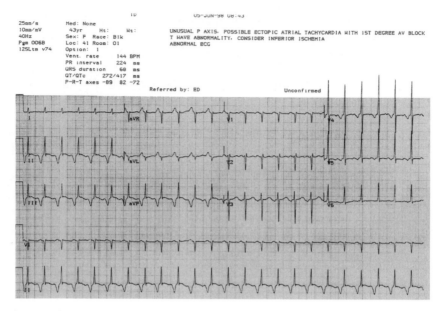

Fig. 4. Atrial tachycardia. This ECG shows a narrow complex tachycardia with deeply inverted P waves most noticeable in the inferior leads. This may be confused with re-entrant tachycardia, except that the PR interval is less than the R-P interval.

and other congenital heart defects leaves the presence of scar tissue in the myocardium [1–5]. This scarred myocardium has rates of conduction and refractoriness that differ from the surrounding myocardium, which allows for a re-entrant loop to be possible. In this setting, a PAC precipitates the onset of the tachycardia loop, which gives it a paroxysmal nature that initiates and stops abruptly. Atrial tachycardias caused by triggered activity are usually seen in the setting of a patient who has a known cardiomyopathy on digoxin. These rhythms tend to be prolonged and are difficult to treat. They are also characterized by a warm-up period at onset and a cool-down period at termination rather than the abrupt nature of re-entrant loops. In digoxin-toxic atrial tachycardias, there is usually an associated AV block (Fig. 5).

The atrial rate is typically 150–250 bpm. Atrial P waves must be seen and should have a different morphology than the P waves in sinus rhythm (see Fig. 4). The morphology of the P wave in leads aVL and V1 may provide clues as to the site of origin. A positive P wave in lead V1 carries a 93% sensitivity and 88% specificity for a left atrial focus. In contrast, a positive or biphasic P wave in lead aVL predicts a right atrial focus with 88% sensitivity and 79% specificity [5].

Junctional tachycardia

This is an uncommon dysrhythmia that usually originates from a discrete focus within the AVN or His bundle. It is a regular, narrow-complex

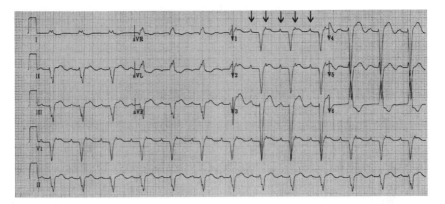

Fig. 5. Atrial tachycardia with AV block. There is evidence of atrial tachycardia at approximately 154 bpm with P waves most noticeable in lead V1 (*arrows*). There is a regular ventricular activity at 77 bpm with a fixed PR interval that indicates this is atrial tachycardia with 2:1 block. The presence of atrial tachycardia with AV block is classic for digoxin toxicity. This may be confused with sinus tachycardia and AV block, yet the clinical setting should support the need for sinus tachycardia, P wave morphology should be identical to baseline, and it is rarely associated with 2:1 AV block.

tachycardia that is caused by enhanced automaticity or triggered activity [6]. As seen in most automatic rhythms, there is usually a warm-up and cool-down phase at initiation and termination. Retrograde activation of the atria does occur, and P′ waves may be seen before or following each QRS complex, although they are usually buried within the QRS complex. The QRS complex is usually narrow, except when there is a pre-existing BBB or a rate-related aberrancy.

Junctional tachycardia is characterized by gradual onset and ventricular rates ranging from 70–130 bpm. That ventricular rates are only slightly faster than sinus rates in this rhythm leading to a common ECG finding of AV dissociation. In this case the AVN is functional, but the junctional pacemaker partially or fully depolarizes the AVN and infranodal tissues, essentially blocking the AVN (Fig. 6).

This rhythm is usually associated with myocardial ischemia/infarction, cardiomyopathy, and digoxin toxicity. In children, particularly infants, this rhythm indicates serious underlying heart disease. It may be confused with atrial fibrillation when retrograde P′ waves are not visible, although the irregularity associated with this rhythm is minor when compared with atrial fibrillation.

Atrial flutter

Atrial flutter is a supraventricular rhythm that is generated by a re-entrant loop just above the AVN in the right atrium. The rate of atrial depolarization created by this circuit is rapid, ranging from 250–350 bpm. The loop usually runs in a counterclockwise direction causing a negative flutter

18

STAHMER & COWAN

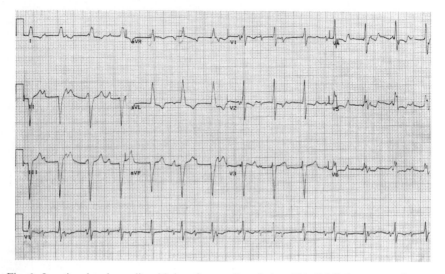

Fig. 6. Junctional tachycardia with interference dissociation. This ECG shows a regular ventricular rhythm between 70 and 100 bpm. There are P waves visible at a rate of 110 bpm, yet they have no clear relationship to the QRS complexes. This is an example of dissociation caused by two competing rhythms—sinus tachycardia and junctional tachycardia—that keep the AVN depolarized.

wave with a downward vector in leads II, III, and aVF. Because the rhythm is generated by a re-entrant loop, the untreated atrial rhythm is regular. The AVN inherently cannot conduct at rates much greater than 200 bpm, and thus not every atrial contraction can generate a ventricular contraction. The ventricular rate therefore is some fraction of the atrial rate (ie, 2:1 or 3:1; atrial rate:ventricular rate). In the absence of AVN disease or medications that act at the AVN, the ventricular rate should be approximately 150 bpm (2:1) or 100 bpm (3:1). Additionally, because the rhythm is a re-entrant one, the rate should be fixed, meaning that there should not be any variation in the rate over time. Atrial flutter that starts at a rhythm of 148 bpm should stay at 148 bpm as long as the patient remains in atrial flutter and has received no medications. Seeing a narrow complex tachycardia on the monitor at a rate of approximately 150 bpm that does not change over time is an important clue to atrial flutter.

Because the circuit is rotating along the base of the atrium, the circuit is always moving toward, then away from, lead II (clockwise or counterclockwise). On the ECG this produces a typical sawtooth pattern seen best in the inferior leads (Fig. 7). The circuit is never running perpendicular to lead II; therefore, on the ECG there is no area in that lead that is isoelectric. If it is difficult to determine the isoelectric point in lead II (usually the T-P interval), the underlying rhythm is suspicious for atrial flutter. When the ventricular response rate is 150 bpm or greater, it can often be difficult to identify the flutter waves. One way to determine the rhythm is to slow the ventricular

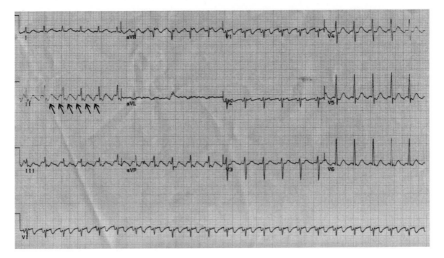

Fig. 7. Atrial flutter. This ECG shows a regular tachycardia at 146 bpm. Inspection of the inferior leads shows the distortion of the ST segment by the flutter waves (*arrows*).

response by way of vagal maneuvers or medications that slow AVN conduction and thus reveal the underlying atrial rhythm. Adenosine is a useful medication in this regard in that it completely blocks the AVN briefly (10–30 sec). When given to a patient in atrial flutter, this undeniably reveals the classic flutter waves as the ventricular rate transiently slows. Because the AVN is not involved in the flutter circuit, adenosine does not terminate the rhythm or serve as long-term treatment.

Paroxysmal supraventricular tachycardia/AVN re-entrant tachycardia

Paroxysmal supraventricular tachycardia/AVN re-entrant tachycardia (AVNRT) comprises 50%–60% of SVTs that are referred for electrophysiologic studies, making it by far the most common type of SVT [1–5]. AVNRT is rhythm that occurs because of a re-entrant loop at the AVN (see Fig. 1). In the AVN, there are usually multiple pathways that are not precisely defined. Most often there are two tracts, one of which is posterior (slow) and one of which is anterior (fast). The anterior tract, used in normal AVN conduction, is characterized by fast transmission through the node and a long refractory period. It is this long refractory period that limits the rate at which the AVN can conduct signals. The posterior tract has the opposite characteristic; it is inherently slower in conducting signals, but has a short refractory period. These rhythms are usually precipitated by a PAC that finds the anterior pathway refractory to antegrade conduction because of its longer refractory period. The posterior pathway is able to conduct down the slow side of the loop because of its shorter refractory period. On reaching the end of the AVN, the fast side is no longer refractory and the signal then travels quickly back up to the top of the AVN. At this point the slow path is ready to conduct and the loop is completed.

The ECG in AVNRT shows a regular rhythm with a ventricular rate that varies from 140–280 bpm (Fig. 8). In the absence of a pre-existing or rate-related BBB, the QRS complex is narrow. Following the initial PAC that is conducted through the slow pathway, the subsequent atrial depolarizations are retrograde. Because retrograde activation is by way of the fast pathway, the P wave is usually buried within the QRS complex. When the P wave is seen, it suggests that the re-entry pathway conducting retrograde is the slow pathway or a bypass tract.

The precipitating event in re-entrant tachycardias is usually a PAC, and so any process that causes PACs puts the patient at risk for development of the rhythm. These include processes that result in atrial stretch (acute coronary syndromes, congestive heart failure), irritability (exogenous catecholamines), and irritation (pericarditis).

Paroxysmal supraventricular tachycardia/orthodromic reciprocating tachycardia

Paroxysmal supraventricular tachycardia/orthodromic reciprocating tachycardia (ORT) comprises approximately 30% of paroxysmal SVTs [7–9]. It usually occurs in patients who are younger in comparison to those with AVNRT. ORT, also known as atrioventricular re-entry tachycardia (AVRT), is similar to AVNRT in that there is a re-entrant loop tachycardia initiated by a PAC. This rhythm, however, is maintained by a different pathway between the atrium and ventricle. In this rhythm, there is antegrade conduction through the normal AVN-His-Purkinje system, as with normal

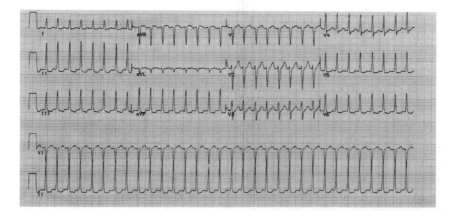

Fig. 8. AVN re-entry tachycardia. This is a regular narrow complex tachycardia without demonstrable P waves. This cannot be atrial flutter, because the rate on this tracing is too slow for 1:1 conduction and too fast for 2:1 (which would be approximately 150 bpm). Administration of adenosine or vagal maneuvers breaks the rhythm and converts to normal sinus rhythm.

sinus rhythm. In contrast to AVNRT, retrograde conduction is by way of an accessory pathway that most often has slow conduction but rapid recovery. The P wave is likely to be visible on the ECG and displaced from the QRS complex (long R-P interval), because the retrograde conduction is through an accessory pathway that is inherently slow in its conduction. Atrial tissue is activated retrograde from the periannular tissue; thus, the P waves are inverted in the inferior leads.

The ECG demonstrates a narrow complex tachycardia with a rate between 140 and 280 bpm (Fig. 9). In general, the rate of ORT tends to be faster than AVNRT. Antegrade conduction occurs by way of the normal AVN conduction system with retrograde conduction by way of a concealed accessory pathway and the QRS complex is narrow. The presence of QRS alternans (alternating amplitude of the QRS complex) has been described in all atrial tachycardias, particularly those that are very fast, but is observed significantly more often in ORT [7,8].

Irregular supraventricular tachydysrhythmias

Multifocal atrial tachycardia

This rhythm typically is seen in patients who have underlying pulmonary disease; it is a narrow complex, irregular tachycardia that is caused by abnormal automaticity of multiple atrial foci. The P waves demonstrate at least three different morphologies in one lead with variable PR intervals. There is no dominant atrial pacemaker. The atrial rate varies from 100–180 bpm. The QRS complexes are uniform in appearance [10] (Fig. 10). This rhythm frequently is mistaken for sinus tachycardia with frequent PACs or atrial fibrillation. The distinguishing feature of multifocal atrial tachycardia is the presence of at least three distinct P wave morphologies in the classic clinical setting of an elderly patient who has symptomatic cardiopulmonary disease. The clinical importance of correctly identifying this rhythm is that treatment should focus on reversing the underlying disease process; rarely is the rhythm responsible for acute symptoms.

Atrial fibrillation

Atrial fibrillation is characterized by a lack of organized atrial activity. The chaotic appearance of this dysrhythmia is caused by the presence of multiple, shifting re-entrant atrial wavelets that result in an irregular baseline that may appear flat or grossly irregular. The rate of atrial depolarization ranges from 400–700 bpm, all of which clearly are not conducted through the AVN. The slow and irregular ventricular response is caused by the requisite AVN recovery times following depolarization and partial conduction of impulses by the AVN, thus rendering it refractory. The ventricular response is irregularly irregular with a rate (untreated) that varies

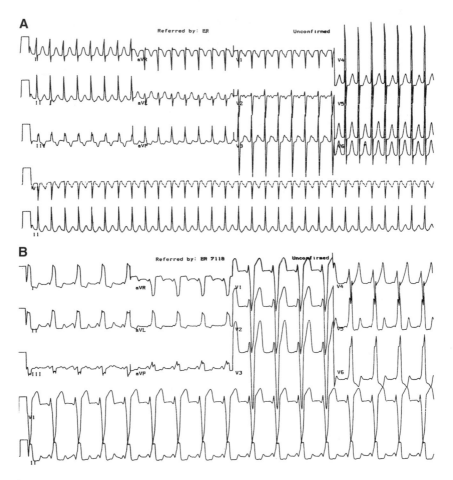

Fig. 9. Orthodromic tachycardia. (*A*) This is a rapid, narrow complex tachycardia that may be virtually indistinguishable from AVNRT until the rhythm breaks, at which time the ECG demonstrates the presence of an accessory pathway as seen in (*B*), with widened QRS complex, delta wave, and shortened PR interval. The ECG in (*A*) reveals an extremely rapid rate, greater than 200 bpm. The narrow QRS complex indicates there is normal antegrade activation of the ventricle by way of the AVN, and AVN blocking agents can be used to break the re-entry circuit.

from 100–200 bpm. Untreated ventricular response rates less than 100 bpm suggest the presence of significant AVN disease, and therapies that increase AVN refractoriness should be administered with caution.

The QRS complex is usually narrow unless there is aberrant conduction or a pre-existing BBB. Aberrant conduction is common in atrial fibrillation because of wide fluctuations in R-R intervals. The underlying mechanism is based on the fact the ventricular recovery is determined by the R-R interval immediately preceding it. When there is a very short R-R interval following a long R-R interval, the ventricle may be refractory and the beat conducted

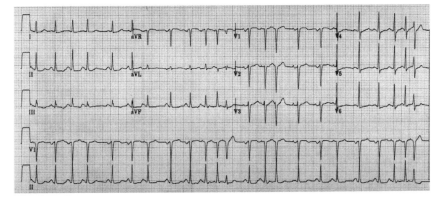

Fig. 10. Multifocal atrial tachycardia. This ECG shows a narrow complex irregular tachydysrhythmia with at least three different P wave morphologies.

aberrantly, termed Ashmann phenomenon. This sometimes can lead to a run of aberrantly conducted beats and may be mistaken for VT (Fig. 11).

Fibrillatory waves have been described as fine or coarse, depending on the amplitude; coarse waves have been associated with atrial enlargement. Atrial fibrillation may be confused with other irregular narrow complex dysrhythmias, such as multifocal atrial tachycardia, atrial tachycardias with variable block, and atrial flutter. The distinguishing feature in atrial fibrillation is the absence of any clear atrial activity; the baseline ECG should be inspected carefully for dominant or repetitive perturbations suggesting uniform atrial depolarizations. Atrial flutter is a macro re-entrant circuit within the right atrium, and the circuitous path of atrial depolarization regularly distorts the ECG baseline. The flutter waves are uniform and regular (see Fig. 7), in contrast to the irregular chaotic activity seen in atrial fibrillation.

Wide complex tachydysrhythmias

The key to differentiating among the various causes of wide QRS complex tachydysrhythmias (WCTs) is the determination of why the complex is wide. Reasons for a wide QRS complex are as follows:

1. There is a pre-existing BBB. In this case the morphology of the QRS complex should look like a typical BBB and review of a prior ECG should demonstrate that the QRS complex morphology is the same. If no prior ECG is available, then familiarity with the characteristic morphology of BBB is crucial. Inspection of the QRS complex in lead V1 is the first step; a principally positive QRS deflection in V1 suggests a right BBB (RBBB) and a principally negative QRS deflection in lead V1 suggests a left BBB (LBBB). In patients who have a positive QRS complex in V1, an RSR' morphology and an Rs wave in V6 with R wave height greater than S wave depth are highly supportive of a pre-existing RBBB.

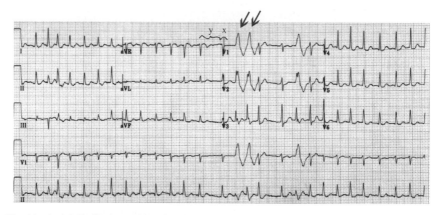

Fig. 11. Atrial fibrillation. This ECG demonstrates an irregular, narrow complex tachycardia. The *arrows* point to aberrantly conducted beats caused by a short coupling (R-R) interval (*x*) following a long coupling interval (*y*). This is referred to as Ashmann aberrancy or Ashmann phenomenon.

In patients who have suspected SVT with LBBB morphology, the presence of an rS or QS wave in leads V1 and V2, delay to S wave nadir of <0.07 seconds, and R wave without preceding Q wave in lead V6 is diagnostic of LBBB (Fig. 12) [11–15].

2. There is a rate-related bundle branch delay or block. Aberrancy occurs when there is slow or absent conduction through the bundle branches. This is observed most often in the setting of abrupt changes in heart rate, most often in atrial fibrillation, but also can be seen in any SVT. The refractory period of the His-Purkinje system depends on the cycle length (the R-R interval) of the beat immediately preceding it. A beat that occurs early or at a distinctly shorter R-R interval may find one bundle partially or completely refractory. The resultant QRS complex manifests a BBB pattern (Fig. 13A,B). The right bundle branch is affected most often and the aberrantly conducted beats have an incomplete or complete RBBB pattern [16–18]. The cause of the tachycardia is supraventricular.

3. The dysrhythmia is originating from the ventricle. The QRS complex is typically wide because the source is distant from the normal activation pathways and ventricular depolarization is prolonged. The QRS complex is wide and has a morphology that is not consistent with a right or left BBB. If the site of activation is near one of the bundles, as in a right ventricular outflow tract tachycardia, the appearance of the QRS complex may be similar to a BBB, but careful inspection of the ECG usually reveals key discrepancies.

4. There is an accessory pathway. In normal sinus rhythm, the usual manifestation of an accessory pathway is premature ventricular activation (the delta wave) with minimal widening of the QRS complex. Depending

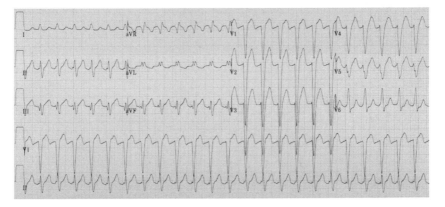

Fig. 12. AVNRT and LBBB. This is a wide complex tachycardia with a QRS complex morphology typical for an LBBB.

on the underlying mechanism, preferential conduction down the accessory pathway distorts and widens the QRS complex. Examples of this include re-entrant dysrhythmias conducting antegrade down the accessory pathway and atrial flutter/fibrillation, where there is preferential conduction down the accessory pathway at faster atrial rates. The rhythm is always supraventricular, and the presence of the accessory pathway alters the pathway of ventricular activation and distorts the QRS complex morphology.

Careful inspection of the ECG can often allow differentiation of these various causes, but it must also be interpreted in the context of the patient and clinical presentation. For example, a WCT presenting in a 55-year-old man with a history of MI is likely to be VT and not the first clinical presentation of an accessory pathway.

Ventricular tachycardia

VT is defined as a series of >3 consecutive wide complex beats with a rate greater than 100 bpm. It is usually regular. Several decision rules have been proposed attempting to identify features on the 12-lead ECG to aid in the diagnosis of VT [19–21]. The criteria vary in their reliability when applied individually and must be interpreted in conjunction with other criteria, the patient's clinical presentation, medical history, and prior ECGs when available.

A frequently used diagnostic algorithm by Brugada incorporates many previously published morphologic criteria in a stepwise algorithm and has been demonstrated to be very sensitive and specific in the absence of pre-existing intraventricular conduction abnormalities (Table 1) [22]. The first step in analyzing the ECG is to determine whether there are any RS complexes in the precordial leads. The presence of RS complexes indicates

A

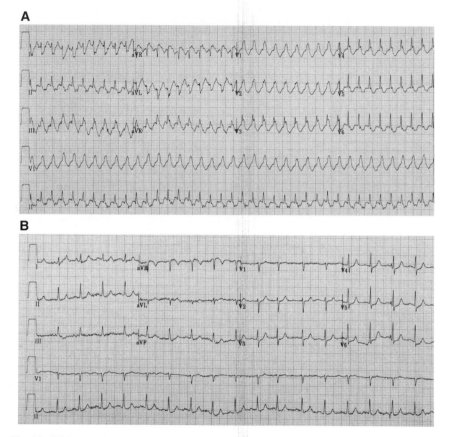

B

Fig. 13. Wide complex tachycardia: rate-related BBB. (*A*) This is a wide complex tachycardia with a QRS complex that demonstrates a typical RBBB appearance. The differential diagnosis includes atrial flutter, AVNRT, and VT. (*B*) Adenosine converted the rhythm to normal sinus rhythm, and the QRS complex morphology was markedly different. Although there was baseline evidence of an incomplete RBBB, the QRS complex is now significantly narrower.

that for the lead in which it was observed, ventricular activation is bidirectional. RS complexes are present in BBB, rate-related aberrancy, and VT. When they are not observed, which is infrequently, the rhythm is likely to be VT (Fig. 14).

The next step is to determine whether the interval from the onset of the R wave to the nadir of the S wave is greater than 0.10 seconds in any precordial leads. This delay typically is not seen in BBB, in which the functioning bundle initiates ventricular activation rapidly with a brisk downstroke (or upstroke) and the electrocardiographic manifestation of the blocked bundle is delays in the terminal portion of the ECG (Fig. 15).

The presence of AV dissociation, another rare finding, is virtually diagnostic of VT. It is useful to examine the ECG carefully for AV dissociation

Table 1
Diagnosis of wide QRS complex tachycardia

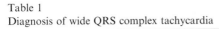

Diagnosis of wide QRS complex tachycardia with a regular rhythm
  Step 1. Is there absence of an RS complex in all precordial leads V1–V6?

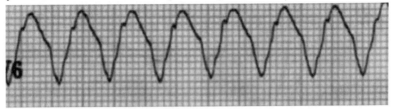

  If yes, then the rhythm is VT.

  Step 2. Is the interval from the onset of the R wave to the nadir
  of the S wave greater than 100 msec (0.10 sec) in any precordial leads?

RS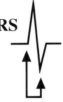

  If yes, then the rhythm is VT.

  Step 3. Is there AV dissociation?
  If yes, then the rhythm is VT.

  Step 4. Are morphology criteria for VT present? See table 2.
  If yes, then the rhythm is VT.

---

when the ventricular rate is slow—faster rates make identification of disso-
ciated P waves particularly difficult. In slower VT, the sinus pacemaker may
have the opportunity to send an impulse at a time when the ventricle is fully
or partially recovered. It may completely or partially depolarize the ventricle
in the normal pattern of activation, resulting in capture or fusion beats, respectively. Capture beats have a morphology identical to that of the ECG in
normal sinus rhythm, whereas fusion beats have a morphologic appearance
that is a fusion of the supraventricular and ventricular pattern of activation
(Figs. 16 and 17).

A final step is to examine the QRS complex morphology and determine
whether the QRS complex most closely resembles a right or left BBB. If
the complex is upright in lead V1 of a standard 12-lead ECG, then it is defined as a right bundle branch type. Although many lead V1-positive VTs
resemble an RBBB, findings indicative of VT include reversal of the normal
rSR′ pattern (to RSr′) and an R/S ratio <1 in V6 (Fig. 18) [21–24]. The latter makes sense if one considers that in RBBB the initial activation of the
ventricle is by way of the left bundle branch and should be manifest as an
initial positive deflection in V6.

Table 2
Morphologic criteria for ventricular tachycardia

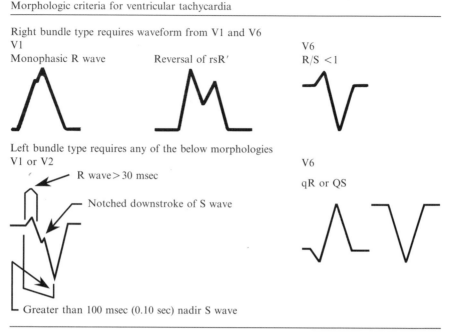

If the complex is negative in lead V1, then it is defined as a left bundle branch type. LBBB morphologies are common in wide complex tachycardias, and close inspection of the QRS morphology and frontal plane QRS axis is helpful in identifying those patients who have VT. Morphologic criteria that can be used to diagnose VT in patients who have lead V1-negative VT are any R in leads V1 or V2 greater than 30 msec (0.03 seconds) in duration, which normally is not seen in SVT with LBBB aberrancy. The presence of any Q wave in lead V6 is also inconsistent with an LBBB and makes sense if one considers that lead V6 "looks" directly at the left ventricle, and activation from a supraventricular site should depolarize the ventricle from the base to the apex, hence toward lead V6. Finally, LBBB aberrancy in SVT, the downstroke of the S wave in lead V1, is usually rapid and smooth. In VT, the duration from the onset of the QRS complex to the nadir of the S wave is often greater than 60 msec (0.06 seconds). The longer the measured duration, the more likely the diagnosis is VT. Further inspection of the S wave also may reveal notching of the downstroke in leads V1 or V2, which is also highly suggestive of VT (see Figs. 14, 15, and 17) [20–24].

Rather than attempt to commit to memory the various morphology types and combinations, inspection of the QRS complex often reveals that morphologies that are inconsistent with a BBB are likely to be VT. Understanding of the typical ECG manifestation of a BBB aids in determining whether the wide complex is typical or not.

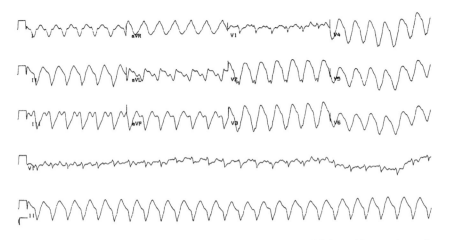

Fig. 14. Wide complex tachycardia with precordial concordance. This is a wide complex tachycardia with a QRS complex morphology that is lead V1-negative, but clearly has little resemblance to an LBBB. There is prolonged duration from onset of R-to-S wave and a QS pattern in lead V6. Additional evidence supporting the diagnosis of VT is the presence of precordial concordance—the QRS complexes point in the same direction as they move across the precordium, ie, there is no QRS complex transition zone. Furthermore, there is a right superior QRS axis (indeterminate axis), which indicates that the site of activation can come only from the ventricular apex.

Polymorphic ventricular tachycardia

Polymorphic VT usually is classified into those rhythms that are associated with prolongation of the QT interval and those with normal baseline QT intervals. Torsades de pointes is a rapid polymorphic VT seen in patients

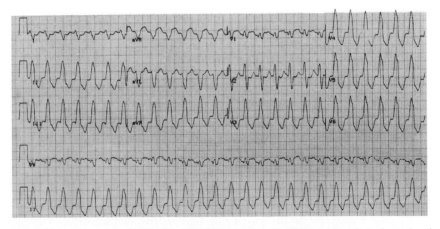

Fig. 15. Ventricular tachycardia. Note the QRS complex morphology; there is prolonged activation from the onset of the R wave to the S wave of more than 0.10 seconds.

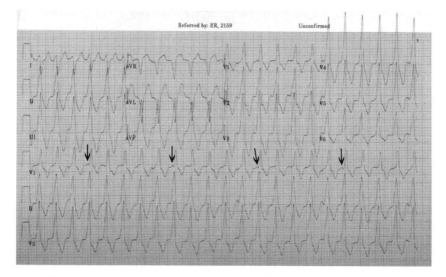

Fig. 16. Ventricular tachycardia with AV dissociation. Although the QRS complex morphology is similar to an RBBB, the presence of AV dissociation indicates this is VT (*arrows* denote regular P waves, although some are lost in the intervening complexes).

who have prolongation of the QT interval; it is characterized by rapidly changing variability in the amplitude and polarity of QRS complexes. The resultant QRS complexes seem to twist around the isoelectric line. A prerequisite for the rhythm is baseline prolongation of the QT interval, which may be congenital or acquired. Torsades de pointes is believed to

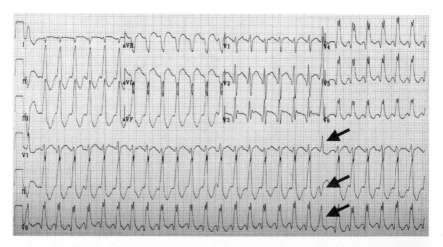

Fig. 17. Wide complex tachycardia. This is a wide complex tachycardia in which the QRS morphology resembles neither LBBB nor RBBB. A fusion beat (*arrow*) is seen in the rhythm strip; its presence confirms VT.

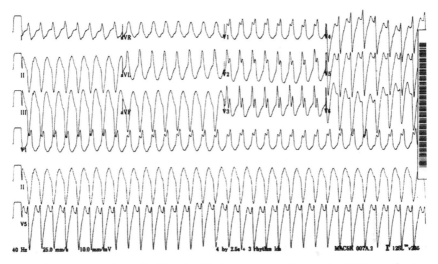

Fig. 18. Ventricular tachycardia. This is VT, showing a lead V1-positive QRS complex morphology that does resemble an RBBB. Closer inspection shows that there is reversal of the rSR' in lead V2 and V3 and an R/S ratio <1 in lead V6, supporting the diagnosis of VT.

arise from early after-depolarizations initiated by a premature ventricular beat or salvo of ventricular beats, followed by a pause and then a supraventricular beat. Another premature ventricular beat arrives at a short coupling interval and falls on the preceding T wave, precipitating the rhythm (Fig. 19) [20–26].

Torsades de pointes is usually paroxysmal in nature and regular, and there are typically 5–20 complexes in each cycle. The ventricular rate is usually 200–250 bpm, and the amplitude of the QRS complexes varies in a sinusoidal pattern. The baseline ECG usually provides important clues to the cause of the dysrhythmia. The presence of a corrected QT interval (QTc) of greater than 0.44–0.45 seconds should be considered abnormal. Patients with QTc intervals greater than 0.50 seconds, and certainly longer than 0.60 seconds, have been shown to be at increased risk for torsades des pointes. In addition to prolongation of the QTc, there may be changes in the ST segment and T wave that would provide clues to an underlying metabolic abnormality.

Polymorphic VT looks like torsades de pointes; the difference is the absence of QT interval prolongation in the baseline ECG. Patients who have this rhythm often are found to have unstable coronary artery disease, and acute myocardial ischemia is believed to be an important prerequisite for this dysrhythmia. These patients are usually unstable, and defibrillation is the treatment of choice.

Polymorphic VT is readily appreciated as a potentially life-threatening rhythm. The only other dysrhythmia that may be easily mistaken for this is atrial fibrillation with a bypass tract. The presence of a bypass tract

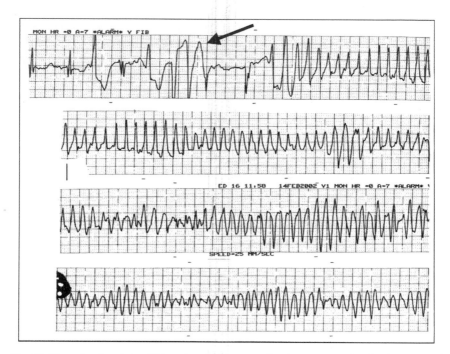

Fig. 19. Torsades de pointes. This series of telemetry strips demonstrates the classic pattern of initiation of this form of polymorphic VT, with a series of early ventricular beats (*arrow*) that fall on the vulnerable period of the prolonged QT interval. These beats are caused by ventricular after-depolarizations that trigger an extrasystole.

that contributes to ventricular depolarization causes the QRS to vary in width and morphology, similar to polymorphic VT. The distinguishing feature of this particular dysrhythmia is that it is grossly irregular because of the underlying rhythm (atrial fibrillation) and the morphology of the QRS complex varies in width and not in amplitude.

Right ventricular outflow tract ventricular tachycardia

This form of VT is seen in patients who do not have underlying heart disease. It originates from or near the right ventricular outflow tract (RVOT) in the interventricular septum and typically has an LBBB morphology and right inferior axis. It is a narrow VT that may be difficult to differentiate from an LBBB. Clues to the origin of the dysrhythmia are characteristic notching in the downslope of the QRS in V1 and, often, breaks in the rhythm that allow for inspection of the baseline ECG (Fig. 20). Patients present with palpitations or syncope, and triggers are believed to be exercise and other causes of increased adrenergic tone. It typically responds to beta-adrenergic or calcium channel blockade. It has been reported to respond to adenosine and as such can be misinterpreted as SVT with aberrancy.

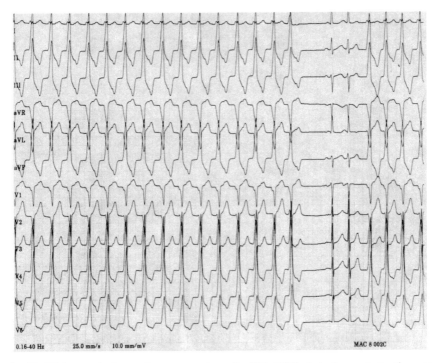

Fig. 20. Right ventricular outflow tract tachycardia. This ECG nicely demonstrates the presence of a wide complex tachycardia that stops abruptly and is followed by narrow complex beats; the first is a sinus beat, whereas the second seems to be a premature supraventricular beat. The typical features of RVOT include the notching in the downstroke of the QRS complex in lead V1, and the QRS complex morphology similar to an LBBB supporting the RVOT activation site.

Accelerated idioventricular rhythm

This rhythm typically is associated with reperfusion in acute MI. It originates in the ventricle and is referred to as accelerated because the ventricular rate, 60–100 bpm, is faster than a ventricular escape rhythm (usually 20–40 bpm), but is not truly tachycardic (ie, > 100 bpm). The QRS complex is regular and wide and the morphology reflects the site of origin, usually having an appearance that is dissimilar to a right or left BBB. This rhythm is usually paroxysmal in nature, lasting less than a minute and allowing for inspection of the underlying ECG. The slow ventricular rate allows for frequent capture or fusion beats (Fig. 21).

Pre-excitation syndromes (Wolff Parkinson White syndrome)

Wolff Parkinson White syndrome (WPW) is a syndrome defined by the presence of an accessory pathway and a predisposition to the development of supraventricular tachydysrhythmias [27]. The presence of the pathway

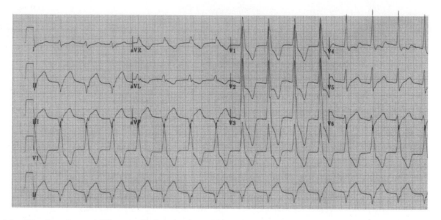

Fig. 21. Accelerated idioventricular rhythm. This is a rhythm that is caused by enhanced automaticity of the Purkinje fibers. It is seen most often in patients who have received thrombolytic therapy and is referred to as a reperfusion dysrhythmia.

not only alters the appearance of the QRS complex during many dysrhythmias but also may affect treatment options with life-threatening implications. Accessory pathways are small bands of tissue that failed to separate during development, allowing continued electrical conduction between the atria and ventricles at sites other than at the AVN. Accessory pathway conduction circumvents the usual conduction delay between the atria and ventricles that occurs within the AVN. This leads to early eccentric activation of the ventricles with subsequent fusion with the usual AVN conduction. The location of the pathway is highly variable and may be situated within free atrial wall connecting to the respective ventricle or in the septum.

For the clinician faced with a patient who has a dysrhythmia involving a bypass tract, the exact location of the tract is not of immediate importance. Of clinical relevance is the ability to recognize that a bypass tract may be present and to appreciate its therapeutic implications. Accessory pathways not only bypass the AVN but also have the capacity to conduct impulses far more rapidly than the AVN. They may conduct antegrade, retrograde, or bidirectionally. A predisposition to tachydysrhythmias is associated with this syndrome, with atrial flutter (5%), atrial fibrillation (10%–20%), and paroxysmal SVT being the most common (40%–80%) [28–30]. Standard treatment of all these dysrhythmias is to increase AVN refractoriness through maneuvers or medications. In the setting of an accessory pathway, these interventions may be ineffective or even deadly, because conduction down the accessory pathway usually is not affected. The role of the accessory pathway in each of these dysrhythmias is discussed briefly in this article.

In patients who have an accessory pathway, the baseline ECG in sinus rhythm may be normal, particularly when the bypass tract is capable of only retrograde conduction. In this case, the presence of the pathway is revealed only in the setting of re-entrant tachydysrhythmias in which the pathway forms the retrograde portion of the re-entrant loop. In patients who have pathways capable of antegrade conduction, the baseline ECG in normal sinus rhythm may show a short PR interval and a delta wave—a slurring of the initial portion of the R wave caused by pre-excitation of the ventricle (Fig. 22). The PR interval is usually less than 0.12 seconds, and the P wave is usually normal in morphology. The QRS complex duration is usually increased because of the presence of the delta wave, and there are secondary repolarization changes seen, manifested as deviation of the ST segment/T wave complex in the direction opposite that of the delta wave and QRS complex (Fig. 23).

The appearance of the QRS complex varies depending on the location of the accessory pathway. WPW has been described by some investigators as type A or type B, depending on the appearance of the delta wave. Type A WPW features a positive, upright delta wave in all precordial leads, and thus has R wave amplitude greater than S wave amplitude in lead V1. In type B, the delta wave and QRS complex are negative in leads V1 and V2 and become positive in the transition to the lateral leads. This pattern closely resembles that of an LBBB. Of note is that even in sinus rhythm there may be variation in the presence and appearance of the delta wave in the same brief rhythm strip and related to the degree of ventricular pre-excitation.

AV re-entrant tachycardia in the presence of an accessory pathway creates a pathway for re-entry dysrhythmias. These are the most common form of tachydysrhythmias associated with WPW and usually are precipitated by a premature atrial or ventricular beat. The re-entrant circuit usually

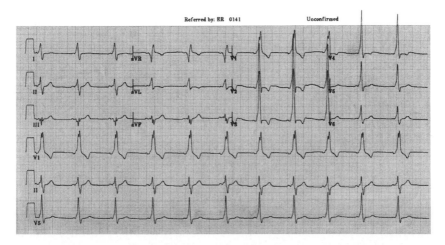

Fig. 22. Wolff Parkinson White syndrome. This ECG demonstrates the typical pattern of early activation of the ventricle by the accessory pathway in normal sinus rhythm.

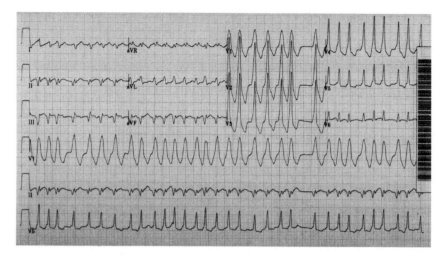

Fig. 23. Wolff Parkinson White syndrome and atrial fibrillation. In atrial fibrillation, the presence of an accessory pathway distorts the QRS complex morphology. The QRS complexes vary on a beat-to-beat basis, which distinguishes it from atrial fibrillation with a pre-existing BBB. An alternative diagnosis would be an SVT with a rate-related BBB, but inspection of the ECG shows that where the R-R interval is the shortest, the QRS complex is actually the narrowest. This is opposite what one would expect from a rate-related BBB, in which faster conduction leads to the aberrancy.

conducts down the AVN and re-enters by way of the accessory pathway. This is referred to as orthodromic tachycardia and appears as a narrow complex, regular tachycardia. The heart rate varies from 140–250 bpm and is generally faster than re-entrant tachycardias that only involve the AVN (see Fig. 9A,B). In a small percentage of patients, the re-entrant circuit conducts antegrade down the accessory pathway and re-enters by way of the AVN. In this case the QRS complex is wide, because all ventricular depolarization is by way of the bypass tract. In both forms of re-entrant tachycardia, the AVN is an integral part of the re-entrant circuit and AVN blocking agents are effective in disrupting the circuit.

Atrial fibrillation and atrial flutter are seen less commonly in association with WPW, and yet are the most feared. In atrial fibrillation and flutter, atrial depolarization rates are equal to or greater than 300 bpm. Atrial impulses normally are blocked, to some extent, at the AVN because of its long refractory period, and ventricular response rates are much slower. Accessory pathways have significantly shorter refractory periods and faster conduction times compared with the AVN, and in these rhythms, nearly all atrial depolarizations are conducted down the accessory pathway. The pattern of ventricular activation varies depending on the relative proportion of electrical activation conducted by way of the AVN and accessory pathway, resulting in widened and bizarre appearing QRS complexes that vary in width on a beat-to-beat basis (Fig. 23).

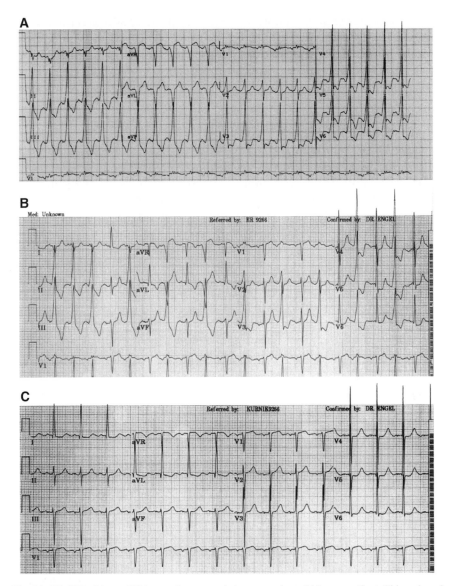

Fig. 24. Wolff Parkinson White syndrome, varied presentation within one patient. This series of ECGs nicely demonstrates the unmasking of an accessory pathway, seen first during sinus tachycardia (*A*). As the heart rate slows (*B*), the sinus beats are alternatively conducted down the bypass tract (wide QRS complex) and the AVN (narrow QRS complex). The pre-excited beats easily could be mistaken for ventricular bigeminy, but closer inspection of the ECG shows that there is a fixed relationship between the P waves (seen best in lead V1) and the wide QRS complexes. As the sinus rate slows still further (*C*), the sinus beats are now conducting solely by way of the AVN, leading to narrow QRS complexes in all beats and a masking of the underlying pre-excitation syndrome.

The appearance of atrial fibrillation in the setting of a bypass tract can be confused easily with polymorphic VT or atrial fibrillation with rate-related aberrancy. The ventricular response in polymorphic VT is never as grossly irregular as atrial fibrillation. Inspection of the ECG in atrial fibrillation with WPW also shows that the QRS complex is usually narrow at the shortest R-R intervals (fastest heart rates) because of sole conduction down the bypass tract. This is because the AVN cannot conduct at ventricular response rates approaching 300 bpm, whereas the bypass tract can. This is in direct contrast to rate-related aberrancy in which the QRS should be most aberrant at the shortest R-R intervals (Fig. 23).

Usual treatment in these rhythms consists of controlling the ventricular rate with agents that block the AVN. In the setting of a bypass tract, blocking the AVN results in impulse conduction entirely down the accessory pathway, which is essentially removing the brakes from the equation. The pathway has the potential to conduct at rates in excess of 300 bpm, which can precipitate degeneration into ventricular fibrillation. In the hemodynamically stable patient, the treatment is to slow conduction through the bypass tract, which traditionally is accomplished with procainamide.

The distortion of the QRS complex by the accessory pathway sometimes can lead to confusion with other dysrhythmias, particularly ventricular rhythms [30]. In the examples shown in Fig. 24A–C, the initial rhythm is a sinus tachycardia with pre-excited beats. This initial rhythm (Fig. 24A) was misinterpreted as accelerated idioventricular rhythm. Clues to the correct diagnosis are the presence of sinus P waves before each beat with a constant, albeit shortened, PR interval. As the sinus rate slows (Fig. 24B), the pre-excited beats occurred intermittently and were misinterpreted as ventricular bigeminy. Further slowing of the sinus rate resulted in disappearance of the pre-excited beats entirely (Fig. 24C).

Summary

Tachydysrhythmias arise from different mechanisms that can be characterized as being caused by re-entrant circuits, enhanced or abnormal automaticity, or triggered after-depolarizations. The approach to the tachydysrhythmia should begin with distinguishing sinus from non-sinus rhythms, then assessing QRS complex width and regularity. Consider the following approach to the ECG demonstrating tachydysrhythmia:

1. Is it a *sinus rhythm*?
2. Is the QRS complex *narrow or wide*?
   a. If the QRS complex is wide, is it regular or irregular?
   b. If the QRS complex is irregular, it is likely not VT, but instead an SVT with pre-existing BBB or rate-related aberrancy; obtain an old ECG if available
   c. If the QRS complex is regular and wide, go through the criteria listed in Table 1

3. If the QRS is *narrow and regular*, it is likely to be:
   a. AVNT or AVRT
   b. Atrial flutter with 2:1 block if the ventricular rate is 130–150 bpm or 1:1 if the rate is 280–340 bpm
   c. Atrial tachycardia—must see P waves
4. If the QRS is *narrow and irregular*, it is likely to be one of the following rhythms:
   a. Atrial fibrillation
   b. Sinus tachycardia with PACs
   c. Multifocal atrial tachycardia
5. Final caveats
   a. Old ECGs are invaluable
   b. Breaks in the rhythms often provide keys to the diagnosis
   c. Response to therapies often confirms or reveals the diagnosis

References

[1] Waldo AL, Wit AL. Mechanisms of cardiac dysrhythmias. Lancet 1993;341:1189–93.
[2] Ferguson JD, DiMarco JP. Contemporary management of paroxysmal supraventricular tachycardia. Circulation 2003;107:1096–9.
[3] Goodacre S, Irons R. Atrial dysrhythmias (clinical review: ABC of clinical electrocardiology). BMJ 2002;324:594–7.
[4] Wathan MS, Klein GJ, Yee R, et al. Classification and terminology of supraventricular tachycardia: diagnosis and management of atrial tachycardias. Cardiol Clin 1993;11: 109–20.
[5] Chauhan VS, Krahn GJ, Skanes AC, et al. Cardiac dysrhythmias-supraventricular tachycardia. Med Clin North Am 2001;85:201–27.
[6] Rosen KM. Junctional tachycardia: mechanisms, diagnosis, differential diagnosis, and management. Circulation 1973;47:654–64.
[7] Trohman RG. Supraventricular tachycardia: implications for the intensivist. Crit Care Med 2000;28(10 Suppl):N129–35.
[8] Green M, Heddle B, Dassan W, et al. Value of QRS alternation in determining the site of origin of narrow QRS supraventricular tachycardia. Circulation 1983;68:368–73.
[9] Kalbfleisch SJ, El-atassi R, Calkins H, et al. Differentiation of paroxysmal narrow QRS complex tachycardias using the 12 lead electrocardiogram. J Am Coll Cardiol 1993;21: 85–9.
[10] Kastor JA. Multifocal atrial tachycardia. N Engl J Med 1990;322:1713–7.
[11] Alberca T, Almendral J, Sanz P, et al. Evaluation of the specificity of morphological electrocardiographic criteria for the differential diagnosis of wide QRS complex tachycardia in patients with intraventricular conduction defects. Circulation 1997;96:3527–33.
[12] Dongas J, Lehmann MH, Mahmud R, et al. Value of preexisting bundle branch block in the electrocardiographic differentiation of supraventricular from ventricular origin of wide QRS tachycardia. Am J Cardiol 1985;55:717–21.
[13] Griffith MJ, Garrett CJ, Mounsey P, et al. Ventricular tachycardia as a default diagnosis in broad complex tachycardias. Lancet 1994;343:386–8.
[14] Coumel P, Leclercq JF, Attuel P, et al. The QRS morphology in post-myocardial infarction ventricular tachycardia. A study of 100 tracings compared with 70 cases of idiopathic ventricular. Eur Heart J 1984;5:792–9.
[15] Brady WJ, Skiles J. Wide QRS complex tachycardia: ECG differential diagnosis. Am J Emerg Med 1999;17:376–81.

[16] Drew BJ, Scheinman MM. ECG criteria to distinguish between aberrantly conducted supraventricular tachycardia and ventricular tachycardia. Practical aspects for the immediate care setting. PACE 1995;18:2194–208.

[17] Pollack ML, Chan TC, Brady WJ. Electrocardiographic manifestations: aberrant ventricular conduction. J Emerg Med 2000;19:363–7.

[18] Betts TR, Goldberger JJ, Kadish AH. Frequency and characteristics of progressive aberrancy during supraventricular tachycardia. Am J Cardiol 2003;92:736–9.

[19] Wellens HJJ, Brugada P. Diagnosis of ventricular tachycardia from the 12-lead electrocardiogram. Cardiol Chin 1987;5:511–25.

[20] Wellens HJJ, Bar FW, Lie KI. The value of the electrocardiogram in the differential diagnosis of a tachycardia with a widened QRS complex. Am J Med 1978;64:27–33.

[21] Kindwall KE, Brown J, Josephson ME. Electrocardiographic criteria for ventricular tachycardia in wide complex left bundle branch block morphology tachycardias. Am J Cardiol 1988;61:1279–83.

[22] Brugada P, Brugada J, Mont L, et al. A new approach to the differential diagnosis of a regular tachycardia with a wide QRS complex. Circulation 1991;83:1649–59.

[23] Akhtar M. Clinical spectrum of ventricular tachycardia. Circulation 1990;82:1561–73.

[24] Munger TM. Ventricular tachycardia electrocardiographic diagnosis (including aberration) and management. In: Murphy JG, editor. Mayo Clinic cardiology review. Futura Publishing Co., Inc.: New York; 1997. p. 457–66.

[25] Gupta AK, Thakur RK. Wide QRS complex tachycardias. Med Clin North Am 2001;85: 245–66.

[26] Passman R, Kadish A. Polymorphic ventricular tachycardia, long Q-T syndrome, and torsades de pointes. Med Clin North Am 2001;85:321–41.

[27] Wolff L, Parkinson J, While PD. Bundle-branch block with short PR interval in healthy young people prone to paroxysmal tachycardia. Am Heart J 1930;5:685–704.

[28] Rosner MH, Brady WJ, Kefer MP, et al. Electrocardiography in the patient with the Wolff-Parkinson-White Syndrome: diagnostic and initial therapeutic issues. Am J Emerg Med 1999;17:705–14.

[29] Bartlett TG, Friedman PL. Current management of the Wolff-Parkinson-White syndrome. J Card Surg 1993;8:503–15.

[30] Wang K, Asinger R, Hodges M. Electrocardiograms of Wolff Parkinson White syndrome simulating other conditions. Am Heart J 1996;132:152–6.

EMERGENCY
MEDICINE
CLINICS OF
NORTH AMERICA

ELSEVIER
SAUNDERS

Emerg Med Clin N Am 24 (2006) 41–51

Intraventricular Conduction Abnormalities

Robert L. Rogers, MD*, MyPhuong Mitarai, MD,
Amal Mattu, MD

*Department of Surgery/Division of Emergency Medicine,
Department of Medicine, Combined Emergency Medicine/Internal Medicine Residency,
University of Maryland School of Medicine, 419 West Redwood Street,
Suite 280, Baltimore, MD 21201, USA*

Intraventricular conduction abnormalities (IVCAs) comprise a group of abnormalities seen on the electrocardiogram (ECG) that often confuse clinicians and may conceal potentially lethal disease entities, such as acute myocardial infarction (MI). Cardiac impulses normally originate in the sinoatrial (SA) node and then are conducted through atrial tissue to the atrioventricular (AV) node and into the bundle of His. Impulses then travel into the right and left bundle branches, which run along the interventricular septum. The right bundle branch remains one fascicle and terminates in Purkinje fibers and then myocardial fibers. The left bundle branches into the left anterior and posterior fascicles. Certain disease processes, such as MI or intrinsic conduction system disease, may affect the conduction system at any point and lead to the development of bundle branch blocks [1]. Bundle branch blocks are just one type of conduction abnormality.

There are multiple types of IVCAs, each with its own unique clinical significance. It is useful to categorize conduction abnormalities, or blocks, by the number of fascicles involved. Unifascicular blocks, such as right bundle branch block (RBBB), left anterior fascicular block (LAFB), and left posterior fascicular block (LPFB), involve a conduction disturbance in one fascicle. Bifascicular blocks, such as left bundle branch block (LBBB), the combination of RBBB and LAFB, or RBBB and LPFB, occur when two of the three fascicles are involved. Finally, trifascicular block denotes a block in all three fascicles. The clinical presentation of IVCAs varies from the asymptomatic patient to the patient in extremis from complete heart block

---

* Corresponding author.
E-mail address: rrogers@medicine.umaryland.edu (R.L. Rogers).

0733-8627/06/$ - see front matter © 2005 Elsevier Inc. All rights reserved.
doi:10.1016/j.emc.2005.08.005   *emed.theclinics.com*

in need of a pacemaker. Intraventricular conduction abnormalities mani-fest on the ECG with the appearance of a widened QRS complex (>0.10 seconds). The common causes of a wide QRS complex are (1) ab-errant ventricular conduction (bundle branch block); (2) ventricular ec-topy/ventricular tachycardia; (3) ventricular paced beats; (4) ventricular pre-excitation syndromes (eg, Wolff Parkinson White syndrome); (5) left ventricular hypertrophy; (6) nonspecific intraventricular conduction delay; (7) hypothermia; (8) hyperkalemia; and (9) drug toxicity (primarily sodium channel blockers, eg, cyclic antidepressants, cocaine).

Unifascicular blocks

Right bundle branch block

RBBB is a common IVCA and is found in patients with and without structural heart disease (Fig. 1). Common causes include MI, hypertensive heart disease, and pulmonary diseases, such as pulmonary embolism and chronic obstructive lung disease. RBBB also can occur in normal individuals without underlying heart disease (Box 1). By definition, the main ECG find-ing in RBBB is a QRS complex duration of 0.12 seconds or greater. Classi-cally, the morphology of the QRS complex in V1 is M-shaped with an rSr′ ("rabbit ear") pattern, but it also can be a single R wave or qR pattern. There is also usually a wide or deep S wave in leads I and V6. Right bundle branch block ECG findings include: (1) widened QRS complex (>0.12 sec-onds), (2) deep, wide S wave in left-sided leads (I, V5, and V6), and (3) sec-ondary R wave in right precordial leads (rsr′, rSR′, or rsR′). With regard to

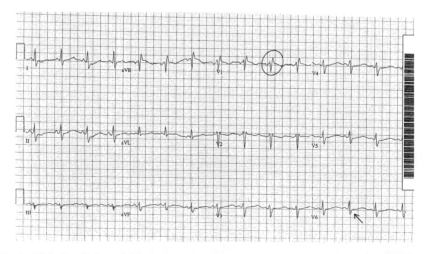

Fig. 1. Right bundle branch block. Note the rSR′ morphology of the QRS complex in lead V1 (*circle*) and the deep, wide S wave in V6 (*arrow*).

Box 1. Differential diagnosis of right bundle branch block

Myocardial infarction
Pulmonary embolism
Chronic obstructive lung disease/cor pulmonale
Pulmonary hypertension (primary or secondary)
Hypertensive heart disease
Degenerative disease of the conduction system
Brugada syndrome
Cardiomyopathy
Chagas disease
Congenital heart disease (eg, Ebstein anomaly)

---

the ST segment/T wave, the ECG typically demonstrates discordance of this complex in the right precordial leads with mild ST segment depression and T wave inversion. ST segment elevation or upright T waves in leads V1–V3 thus suggests the presence of ischemia. If the ECG features of RBBB are found with a QRS complex <0.12 seconds it is referred to as an incomplete right bundle branch block (IRBBB), or a right-sided conduction delay [1].

RBBB can be seen in patients who have pulmonary embolism, with as many as 67% showing evidence of a complete or incomplete right bundle branch block [2]. Given this association, strong consideration for pulmonary embolism should be given to any patient who presents with cardiopulmonary symptoms with evidence of a new (or not known to be old) complete or incomplete RBBB. In a study of 20 cases of centrally-located pulmonary embolism documented by autopsy, 10 patients had RBBB and an additional 6 had IRBBB [2,3]. In the same study, patients with peripheral clots did not manifest an RBBB pattern.

RBBB may occur in patients who have acute MI and is estimated to occur in 3%–7% of patients [4]. The Framingham study has shown that the presence of a new RBBB after previously having had a normal ECG is suggestive of organic heart disease [5]. Coronary artery disease is among many causes of a new RBBB.

The Brugada syndrome is a unique and recently described clinical and electrocardiographic disease entity characterized by an incomplete or complete right bundle branch block pattern and ST segment elevation in the right precordial leads (V1–V3). The underlying pathophysiology is believed to be a defect in the cardiac sodium channel. Brugada and colleagues first described the syndrome in the early 1990s [6]. Its significance lies in that the main cause of death in individuals with the syndrome is sudden cardiac death caused by ventricular tachycardia. Detection of the syndrome is essential in that placement of an automated implantable cardiac defibrillator (AICD), the treatment of choice, is associated with a 100% survival rate.

Without the AICD, mortality is estimated at 10% per year. Emergency physicians should consider this entity in all patients who have a new incomplete or complete RBBB, especially if ST elevation in leads V1–V3 is present. These patients should be referred for electrophysiologic testing for confirmation of the diagnosis. It should be noted that patients who have the Brugada syndrome may be completely asymptomatic or may present after a syncopal episode or in cardiac arrest.

Left anterior fascicular block

In the normal conducting system, cardiac impulses travel down into the left and right bundle branches. The left bundle is further subdivided into anterior and posterior fascicles. Any disease process that interrupts conduction through the anterior fascicle produces a left anterior fascicular block (LAFB) pattern on the surface ECG. LAFB is found in patients with and without structural heart disease and in isolation is of no prognostic significance [1,7]. It is, however, one of the most common intraventricular conduction abnormalities in patients who have acute anterior MI and is found in 4% of cases [8]. When LAFB occurs newly in the presence of an anterior MI, there is a slightly increased risk for progression to advanced heart block. The most common vessel involved in this setting is typically the left anterior descending artery [8].

The ECG findings of LAFB (Fig. 2) include a QRS complex generally <0.12 seconds, a leftward axis shift (usually −45° to −90°), rS pattern in the inferior leads (II, III, and aVF), and qR pattern in leads I and aVL. There is also a delayed intrinsicoid deflection in lead aVL (>0.045 seconds) [9].

Left posterior fascicular block

If disease processes interfere with conduction through the posterior fascicle, a left posterior fascicular block (LPFB) becomes manifest on the ECG

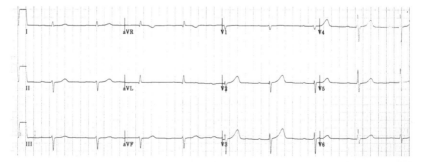

Fig. 2. Left anterior fascicular block. This ECG with sinus bradycardia and a first-degree atrioventricular block also demonstrates left anterior fascicular block. Note the left QRS axis deviation (−60° to −90°), the rS morphology in leads II, III, and aVF, and the small Q wave preceding a larger R wave in leads I and aVL.

(Fig. 3). This particular IVCA is much less common than LAFB [1]. The posterior fascicle has a dual blood supply and is less vulnerable to ischemia than the anterior fascicle. The finding of LPFB is nonspecific and rare [7]. It is found most commonly in patients who have coronary artery disease but can be found in patients who have hypertension and valvular disease. It is reportedly the least common conduction block found in patients who have acute MI [7].

Electrocardiographic findings in LPFB include a rightward axis shift, an rS pattern in leads I and aVL, and a qR pattern in lead III and often in lead aVF. The QRS complex duration is usually normal [1,2].

Bifascicular blocks

Bifascicular block is the combination of an RBBB and an LAFB, or an RBBB plus an LPFB. In addition, because the left bundle branch is composed of an anterior and a posterior fascicle, LBBB can be thought of as a bifascicular block. Bifascicular blocks are of particular importance in the setting of an acute MI, because their presence may suggest impending complete heart block.

The most common type of bifascicular block is the combination of an RBBB and an LAFB (Fig. 4), which occurs in 1% of hospitalized patients [9]. The ECG is characterized by features of an RBBB (QRS duration >0.12 seconds, rsR' or qR in leads V1 and V2, wide or deep S waves in leads I and V6), in addition to a leftward QRS axis and the findings of LAFB (see earlier discussion) in the limb leads. In contrast to the left anterior fascicle, the left posterior fascicle is thicker in structure and has a dual

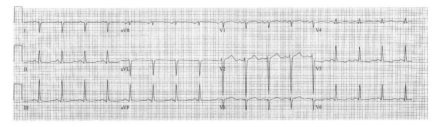

Fig. 3. Left posterior fascicular block. The hallmarks of this rare intraventricular conduction delay are seen here: rightward deviation of the QRS axis (+120°), rS pattern in leads I and aVL, and qR pattern in leads II, III, and aVF. Were there not a small R wave preceding the dominant negative QRS deflection in leads I and aVL (making that an S wave, rather than a QS wave), this would be consistent with a high lateral Q wave myocardial infarction, age indeterminate. Right ventricular hypertrophy should be considered when the ECG seems to show left posterior fascicular block, as both can yield rightward QRS axis deviation. There is no other evidence of right ventricular hypertrophy on this tracing, however (eg, no prominent R wave in lead V1, no prominent S wave in lead V6, and no evidence of right atrial enlargement). At times, echocardiography is needed to exclude definitively right ventricular hypertrophy.

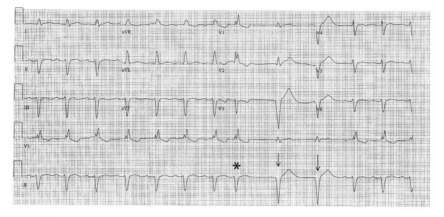

Fig. 4. Right bundle branch block/left anterior fascicular block. Significant leftward deviation of the QRS axis in the presence of right bundle branch block (rsR′ pattern seen in lead V1 plus the deep, wide S wave in lead V6) should lead to consideration of coexistent left anterior fascicular block. Indeed, the rS pattern in the inferior leads together with the qR pattern in the lateral limb leads clinches that diagnosis. There is also a first-degree atrioventricular block (PR interval = 0.21 sec). The ninth and tenth ventricular complexes (*arrows*) following the premature eighth beat (*asterisk*) are ventricular escape complexes.

blood supply; hence, a block of the left posterior fascicle rarely exists by itself. It appears more commonly in conjunction with an RBBB. The ECG findings of an RBBB and an LPFB (Fig. 5) will demonstrate findings of an RBBB, plus a right axis deviation and the other findings of LPFB (see

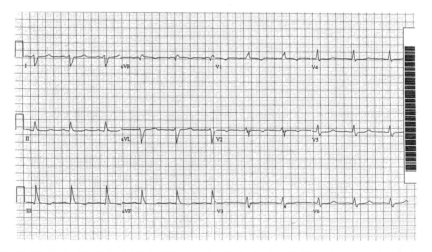

Fig. 5. Right bundle branch block/left posterior fascicular block. Note the rR′ pattern in lead V1 and wide S wave in lead V6—consistent with right bundle branch block. The limb leads demonstrate rightward QRS axis deviation, with an rS pattern in leads I and aVL and the qR pattern in lead III—all consistent with left posterior fascicular block.

earlier discussion). When LPFB does exist, coronary artery disease, hypertensive disease, or aortic valvular disease are common etiologies [10].

Left bundle branch block

A delay in conduction of cardiac impulses through the anterior and posterior fascicles leads to ECG manifestations of LBBB. In this situation, electrical activation of the left ventricle occurs by impulses traveling through the normal right bundle and through the interventricular septum. The most common causes of LBBB include coronary artery disease, hypertension, and cardiomyopathy. Other more rare causes include Lev disease (sclerosis of the cardiac skeleton), Lenegere disease (primary degenerative disease of the conduction system), advanced rheumatic heart disease, and calcific aortic stenosis. An iatrogenic cause of LBBB is produced during cardiac pacing, because the pacing wire usually abuts the right ventricle and induces an LBBB-like morphology on the ECG. The differential diagnosis of left bundle branch block includes: (1) coronary artery disease, (2) cardiomyopathy, (3) hypertensive heart disease, and (4) degenerative disease of the conduction system. The presence of LBBB portends a poor long-term prognosis—one study showed that 50% of patients who have an LBBB die of a cardiac event within 10 years [11].

ECG criteria for LBBB include a QRS duration >0.12 seconds, a broad monomorphic R wave in leads I, V5, and V6, a wide S wave following an initial small (or absent) R wave in the right precordial leads, and absence of septal Q waves in leads I, V5, and V6 (Fig. 6). The term incomplete LBBB is used to describe these findings in patients who have a QRS complex duration <0.12 seconds (usually 0.10–0.11 seconds) Left bundle branch block ECG findings include (1) widened QRS complex (>0.12 seconds), (2) QS or rS complex in lead V1, (3) late intrinsicoid deflection and monophasic R wave in lead V6, and (4) no Q wave in lead V6 [5].

Trifascicular blocks

Trifascicular conduction blocks occur when all three fascicles are involved or if one is permanently blocked and the other two have intermittent conduction delay. Complete trifascicular block can present as a bifascicular block plus a third-degree AV block (Fig. 7). If the block in one of the fascicles is incomplete, the ECG generally demonstrates a bifascicular block and a first- or second-degree AV block. This ultimately can lead to complete heart block. Patients who have multi-fascicular block have advanced conduction system disease that ultimately may progress to complete heart block and sudden cardiac death. The cumulative 3-year rate of sudden death in patients who have bifascicular blocks has been estimated to be 35% in patients who have LBBB, 11% in patients who have RBBB + LAFB, and 7% in

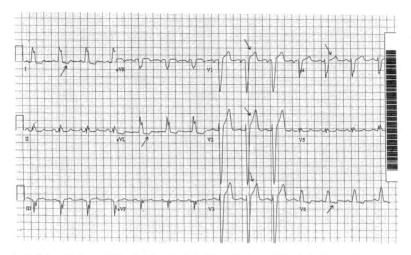

Fig. 6. Left bundle branch block. The classic left bundle branch block findings of a wide (>0.12 sec) monophasic R wave in leads I and V6, rS pattern in leads V1–V3 (here extending to lead V4), and absence of a q wave in lead V6 are all evident on this ECG. The discordant ST segment/T wave complex (ie, opposite to the major vector of the QRS complex [*arrows*]) across the precordial leads (and in leads I and aVL also) is also typical of left bundle branch block.

patients who have RBBB + LPFB [12]. Based on the Framingham study and several other studies performed in the early 1980s, it has been estimated that approximately 1% of patients per year with bifascicular block may progress to complete heart block [11,13].

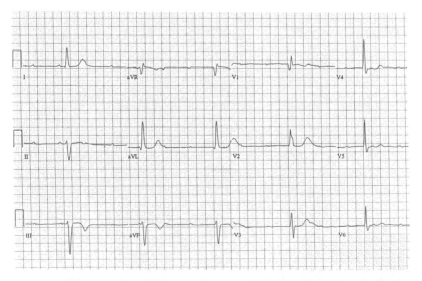

Fig. 7. Trifascicular block. This ECG features right bundle branch block, left anterior fascicular block, and third-degree atrioventricular block (complete heart block).

Rate-dependent bundle branch blocks

Development of right or left bundle branch blocks may be in some cases a rate-related phenomenon [1]. As tachycardia develops, the particular bundle branch block thus becomes evident. Rate-dependent bundle branch block also can occur at slow heart rates. Because tachycardic rate-dependent bundle branch block can simulate ventricular tachycardia or pre-excitation, caution should be exercised when interpreting these electrocardiograms.

Acute myocardial infarction and bundle branch block

In patients who have suspected myocardial ischemia or infarction, the ECG is of paramount importance in helping to determine which patients may need immediate coronary reperfusion. Some of the common ECG findings of myocardial ischemia/infarction include T wave inversion, ST segment depression or elevation, and Q waves. What has been known for many years is that typical ECG findings of a transmural acute MI may be masked in the setting of an LBBB. Although bundle branch blocks are not an independent predictor of mortality, the presence of transient or persistent bundle branch block with acute MI is a recognized marker of increased mortality. In one study, mortality rates for coexistent acute MI and RBBB was shown to be 13.3%, 17% for acute MI and LBBB, and 9.1% for acute MI patients without evidence of a bundle branch block. The Framingham study observed more than 5000 patients for 18 years and found that 1% had new-onset LBBB and that 89% of these patients ultimately suffered a fatal cardiovascular event within several years [4]. Fortunately there is evidence that early administration of fibrinolytic therapy in this group of patients significantly lowers mortality rates if used in the appropriate setting. In a study of more than 800 patients, Brilakis and colleagues [14] found that this population of patients was less likely to receive primary reperfusion therapy, beta-adrenergic blockers, or heparin, and thus was more likely to have higher postdischarge mortality compared with those without an underlying bundle branch block. Survival rates at 1 and 3 years ranged from 56%–80% in patients who had bundle branch block versus 85%–92% in patients without it. On further analysis, primary reperfusion therapy was given to only 13.7% of patients who had bundle branch block versus 31.8% of those without bundle branch blocks [14]. Despite the higher baseline mortality, this population of patients who have bundle branch block and acute MI tend to receive the greatest survival benefit when identified and treated appropriately with fibrinolytic therapy. In 1994, the Fibrinolytic Therapy Trialists reviewed nine major randomized clinical trials of fibrinolytic therapy versus placebo to patients who had bundle branch blocks or acute MI. The benefit of fibrinolytic therapy was observed in patients regardless of age, sex, blood pressure, heart rate, or prior history of infarction or diabetes mellitus, and was greatest with earlier treatment [15].

Right and left bundle branch blocks are seen in 3%–7% and 2%–4% of cases of acute MI, respectively [4]. In general, the interpretation of an ST segment elevation MI (STEMI) is not hindered by the presence of RBBB, because RBBB does not interfere with the direction of septal depolarization or the order of ventricular depolarization. ECG signs of acute MI (ST segment elevation) in the presence of an LBBB may be more obscure and even concealed, contributing to its worse prognosis. In LBBB, conduction crosses the septum in the opposite direction (right-to-left) and depolarizes the ventricles in the reverse order, thus interfering with the initial vectors of ventricular depolarization and obscuring the ECG findings typical of an acute STEMI [16].

In 1996, criteria were developed by Sgarbossa and colleagues from data in the GUSTO-1 database to help aid in diagnosing STEMI in the setting of LBBB. The Sgarbossa criteria for acute ST segment myocardial infarction with coexisting left bundle branch block are (1) ST segment elevation ≥1 mm concordant to QRS complex; (2) ST segment depression ≥1 mm in leads V1, V2, or V3 (concordant to QRS complex); and (3) ST segment elevation ≥5 mm discordant to QRS complex. The criteria include ST segment elevation ≥1 mm in the same direction (concordant) with the QRS complex, ST segment depression ≥1 mm in leads V1, V2, or V3, or ST segment elevation ≥5 mm in the opposite direction (discordant) with the QRS complex; these criteria performed best while maintaining a 90% specificity [17]. A retrospective study by Kontos and colleagues, however, found the Sgarbossa criteria were present in only 3% of 372 patients with LBBB and ischemia [18]. Although the Sgarbossa criteria have been criticized for being too insensitive to use as a screening tool for STEMI in the presence of LBBB, they have been shown to be highly specific and can be used with confidence to confirm acute MI in patients who have LBBB.

References

[1] Mirvis DM, Goldberger AL. Electrocardiography. In: Braunwald E, Zipes DP, Libby P, editors. Heart disease: a textbook of cardiovascular medicine. 6th edition. Philadelphia: WB Saunders; 2001. p. 82–125.
[2] Chan TC, Vilke GM, Pollack MP, et al. Electrocardiographic manifestations: pulmonary embolism. J Emerg Med 2001;21:263–70.
[3] Petrov D. Appearance of right bundle branch block in electrocardiograms of patients with pulmonary embolism as a marker for obstruction of the main pulmonary trunk. J Electrocardiol 2001;34:185–8.
[4] Scheidt S, Killip T. Bundle branch block complicating acute MI. JAMA 1972;222:919–24.
[5] Schneider JF, Thomas HE, Kreger BE, et al. Newly acquired right bundle branch block: the Framingham study. Ann Intern Med 1980;92:37–44.
[6] Brugada P, Brugada J. Right bundle branch block, persistent ST elevation and sudden cardiac death: a distinct clinical and electrocardiographic syndrome. A multicenter report. J Am Coll Cardiol 1992;20:1391–6.

[7] Surawicz BS, Knilans TK. Chou's electrocardiography in clinical practice. 5th edition. Philadelphia: WB Saunders Co; 2001.

[8] Assali A, Sclarovsky S, Herz I, et al. Importance of left anterior hemiblock development in inferior wall acute MI. Am J Cardiol 1997;79:672–4.

[9] Harrigan RA, Pollack ML, Chan TC. Electrocardiographic manifestations: bundle branch blocks and fascicular blocks. J Emerg Med 2003;25(1):67–77.

[10] Braunwald E. Heart disease: a textbook of cardiovascular medicine. 6th edition. Philadelphia: WB Saunders Company; 2001.

[11] Schneider JF, Thomas HE Jr, Kreger BE, et al. Newly acquired left bundle branch block. The Framingham Study. Ann Intern Med 1980;92:37.

[12] Denes P, Dhingra RC, Wu D, et al. Sudden death in patients with chronic bifascicular block. Arch Intern Med 1997;137:1005–10.

[13] McAnulty JH, Rahimtoola SH, Murphy E, et al. Natural history of high risk bundle branch block. Final report of a prospective study. N Engl J Med 1982;307:137.

[14] Brilakis ES, Wright RS, Kopecky SL, et al. Bundle branch block as a predictor of long-term survival after acute MI. Am J Cardiol 2001;1(88):205–9.

[15] Fibrinolytic Therapy Trialists (FTT) Collaborative Group. Indications for fibrinolytic therapy in suspected acute MI: collaborative overview of early mortality and major morbidity results from all randomized trials of more than 1000 patients. Lancet 1994;343:311–22.

[16] Gallagher EJ. Which patients with suspected myocardial ischemia and left bundle branch block should receive thrombolytic agents? Ann Emerg Med 2001;37(5):439–44.

[17] Sgarbossa EB, Pinski SL, Barbagelata A, et al. Electrocardiographic diagnosis of evolving acute MI in the presence of left bundle branch block. GUSTO-I (Global Utilization of Streptokinase and Tissue Plasminogen Activator for Occluded Coronary Arteries) Investigators. N Engl J Med 1996;334:481–7.

[18] Kontos MC, McQueen RH, Jesse RL, et al. Can MI be rapidly identified in emergency department patients who have left bundle branch block? Ann Emerg Med 2001;37:431–8.

ELSEVIER
SAUNDERS

EMERGENCY
MEDICINE
CLINICS OF
NORTH AMERICA

Emerg Med Clin N Am 24 (2006) 53–89

Acute Coronary Syndromes

Stephen W. Smith, MD[a,b,*], Wayne Whitwam, MD[c]

[a]Department of Emergency Medicine, Hennepin County Medical Center, 701 Park Avenue,
Minneapolis, MN 55415, USA
[b]University of Minnesota School of Medicine, 701 South Park Avenue,
Mailcode R-2, Minneapolis, MN 55415, USA
[c]Division of Cardiology, Department of Internal Medicine, University of California,
200 W. Arbor Drive, San Diego 92103-8411, USA

Despite technologic advances in many diagnostic fields, the 12-lead ECG remains the basis for early identification and management of an acute coronary syndrome (ACS). Complete occlusion of coronary arteries (>90%) alters the epicardial surface electrical potentials and usually manifests as ST segment elevation (STE) in two or more adjacent leads. STE may range from <1 mm in a single lead to massive STE as great as 10 mm in multiple leads. This injury pattern represents a myocardial region at risk for (irreversible) myocardial infarction (MI). Such an injury pattern usually leads to at least some myocardial cell death (measured by troponin elevation) and is called ST elevation myocardial infarction (STEMI). STEMI indicates the potential for a substantial irreversible infarction (large risk area) and is the primary indication for emergent reperfusion therapy to salvage myocardium.

In ACS, the elevation of biomarkers (eg, troponin) without *recorded* STE indicates myocardial cell death, but not necessarily that which should be treated with urgent reperfusion therapy. This acute MI (AMI) without STE, though usually with ST segment depression (STD) or T-wave changes, is referred to as non-STEMI (NSTEMI). Unstable angina (UA) implies fully reversible ischemia without troponin release, and its initial clinical and ECG presentation is frequently indistinguishable from NSTEMI. Symptoms of UA are often brief, whereas symptoms of AMI are usually of at least 20 minutes duration; however, patients with 48 hours of symptoms may have UA and those with 5 minutes of symptoms, or none at all, may suffer from NSTEMI. UA and NSTEMI result from a nonocclusive thrombus, small risk area, brief occlusion (spontaneously reperfused), or an occlusion

---

* Corresponding author.
E-mail address: smith253@umn.edu (S.W. Smith).

0733-8627/06/$ - see front matter © 2005 Elsevier Inc. All rights reserved.
doi:10.1016/j.emc.2005.08.008
emed.theclinics.com

that maintains good collateral circulation. In many such cases, there would have been STE, or other ST segment or T-wave abnormalities, had an ECG been recorded at the appropriate time. Similarly, the presence of troponin elevation does not necessarily imply *ongoing* injury or ischemia; this is one reason that the recorded ECG may be normal in AMI. UA and NSTEMI do not require emergent percutaneous coronary intervention (PCI), but PCI within 48 hours reduces the morbidity and mortality of UA/NSTEMI [1].

Many patients who have STEMI who are eligible for emergent reperfusion therapy still do not receive it; this is largely because of difficulties in ECG interpretation, including subtle STE, STE in few leads, and left bundle branch block (LBBB) [2–6]. Patients who have AMI with subtle or nondiagnostic ECGs and atypical symptoms are most likely to be overlooked for reperfusion therapy. Up to 4% are discharged mistakenly from the emergency department, many because of misread ECGs, and they have a high mortality [7–10]. One third of patients diagnosed with AMI, including STEMI, present to emergency departments without chest pain [11]. It is important to record an ECG even in the presence of nonspecific or vague symptoms, and when the ECG is unequivocally diagnostic for STEMI, to act on the ECG despite even atypical symptoms.

Approximately half of AMI, as diagnosed by creatine kinase—MB (CK-MB), manifest clearly diagnostic STE [12–14]. This percentage is less in the era of troponin-defined diagnosis. Much AMI with subtle STE, however, goes unrecognized. Furthermore, most STE result from non-AMI etiologies (eg, left ventricular hypertrophy, acute pericarditis, early repolarization, LBBB, and so on) [15–17]. There are thus false positives and false negatives. With such ECGs, the interpretation must be considered in the context of pretest probability of AMI (ie, the clinical presentation) and by recognition of ECG patterns that mimic AMI [18].

Normal or nondiagnostic ECG as manifestation of non-ST elevation myocardial infarction

A normal initial ECG does not preclude the diagnosis of AMI. Combining two studies, approximately 3.5% of patients who had undifferentiated chest pain and a normal ECG were later diagnosed with AMI by CK-MB, and 9% of such patients who had a nonspecific ECG had an AMI [14,19]. A normal ECG recorded during an episode of chest pain, however, makes ACS a less likely etiology of chest pain, and when ACS is the etiology a normal ECG is associated with a better prognosis [20]. Many additional patients who have normal or nondiagnostic ECGs may have UA. Those who have suspected ACS with a nondiagnostic ECG have fewer in-hospital complications as long as subsequent ECGs remain negative [21,22]. Among patients who have chest pain subsequently diagnosed with AMI by CK-MB, 6% [23] to 8% [14,24,25] have normal ECGs and 22% [26] to 35% [14,19,26] have nonspecific ECGs. There is associated relative mortality risk for AMI even with a normal ECG (0.59) or a nonspecific ECG (0.70) when compared with a diagnostic ECG [26]. These figures are not surprising, especially considering that the coronary plaque is unstable and that many normal or nondiagnostic ECGs are recorded at a temporary moment of adequate perfusion. Accordingly, the sensitivity of the ECG for AMI, including STEMI, is greatly improved with the use of serial ECGs or ST segment monitoring in patients at high clinical suspicion [27]. Furthermore, prehospital tracings often reveal STE that is no longer present in the ED [28].

Evolution of ST elevation myocardial infarction

Within minutes of a coronary occlusion, if recorded on the ECG, hyperacute T waves may manifest, followed by STE (Fig. 1). If the occlusion persists, Q wave formation may begin within 1 hour and be completed by 8–12 hours (representing completed MI) [29]. STE that has peaked rapidly begins to fall slowly as irreversible infarction completes. Shallow T-wave inversion develops within 72 hours; stabilization of the ST segment usually within 12 hours [30], with or without full ST segment resolution over the ensuing 72 hours [31]. T waves may normalize over days, weeks, or months [32]. STE completely resolves within 2 weeks after 95% of inferior and 40% of anterior MI; persistence for more than 2 weeks is associated with greater morbidity [31]. Approximately 60% of patients who have MI with persistent ST segment displacement have an anatomic ventricular aneurysm [31].

Hyperacute T waves

Prominent T waves associated with the earliest phase of STEMI are termed hyperacute T waves (Figs. 2–4). Experimentally, these bulky and wide T waves, often with a depressed ST takeoff (see Fig. 3B and 4) [33,34], are localized to the area of injury and may form as early as 2 minutes after coronary ligation but typically present within the first 30 minutes

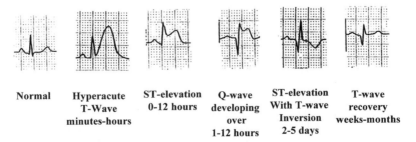

| Normal | Hyperacute T-Wave minutes-hours | ST-elevation 0-12 hours | Q-wave developing over 1-12 hours | ST-elevation With T-wave Inversion 2-5 days | T-wave recovery weeks-months |

Fig. 1. Evolution of inferior STEMI, lead III. *Reprinted with permission from* Wang K. Atlas of electrocardiography.

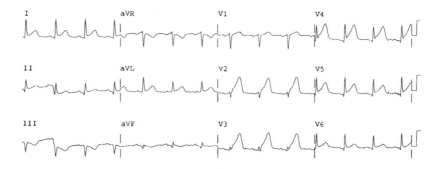

Fig. 2. Hyperacute T waves. Proximal LAD occlusion manifesting hyperacute T waves in addition to ST elevation.

following a clinical event [35–43]. This short-lived ECG feature rapidly progresses to STE and usually is bypassed in actual clinical situations. Even after STE develops, however, the T wave remains prominent (and often hyperacute), and the height of the T wave correlates with the acuteness of the injury. Even at this early phase, there is only subendocardial ischemia without cellular injury. Hence, there may be no associated elevation of troponin [44]. As hyperacute T waves are a marker of early occlusion,

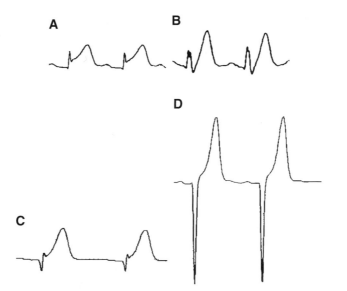

Fig. 3. Four examples of hyperacute T waves. (*A*) Lead V4, T wave is very large compared with QRS. (*B*) Lead V3, with depressed ST segment take-off and straightening of the ST segment. (*C*) wide and bulky, much larger than QRS. (*D*) This less common form is very peaked and tented, with an appearance of hyperkalemia. *Reprinted with permission from* Chan TC, Brady WJ, Harrigan RA, et al. ECG in emergency medicine and acute care. Elsevier; 2005.

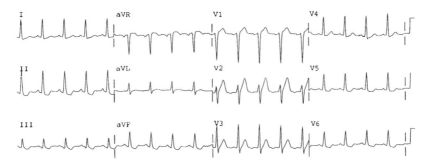

Fig. 4. Early left anterior descending (LAD) occlusion. The most obvious abnormality is diffuse STD in inferior and lateral leads, though there is STE in V1. There is also straightening of ST segments in leads V2 and V3, with slightly large T waves. The patient arrested moments later. He survived after prolonged resuscitation and percutaneous coronary intervention.

reperfusion therapy begun while T waves are prominent correlates with better outcomes [45–48]. The sequence is reversible: if occlusion is brief, hyperacute T waves may be the last abnormality seen on a normalizing ECG after resolution of STE (Fig. 5).

ST segment elevation

STE should be measured from the upper edge of the PR segment (not the TP segment) to the upper edge of the ST segment at the J point; similarly, ST segment depression should be measured from the lower edge of the PR segment to the lower edge of the ST segment, also at the J point. If the ST segment is measured relative to the TP segment, atrial repolarization with a prominent negative Ta wave representing repolarization of the atrium results in an inaccurate measurement. Results are different between measurement at the J point versus 60 ms after the J point [49–52]. On the other hand, STE with a tall T wave, versus without, is much more suggestive of AMI, and measurement at 80 ms after the J point, where the ST segment is slurring up into a tall T wave, reflects the presence of a tall T wave better than measurement at the J point. Measurements are more important for research protocols, however, than for diagnosis of individual patients: a well-informed subjective interpretation of the appearance of the ST segment is more accurate than measured criteria [53,54].

To diagnose STEMI, STE must be new or presumed new. Various clinical trials of thrombolytic therapy have required different STE criteria: for voltage (1 or 2 mm [0.10 or 0.20 mV]) and for the number of leads required (1 or 2 leads) [55–62]. To obtain consistency, a consensus statement defined STEMI as ST segment elevation at the J point, relative to the PR segment, in two or more contiguous leads, with the cut-off points ≥0.2 mV (2 mm) in leads V1, V2, or V3 and ≥0.1 mV (1 mm) in other leads (contiguity in the frontal plane is defined by the lead sequence aVL, I, inverted aVR, II, aVF,

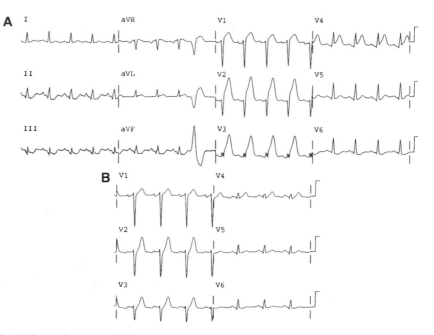

Fig. 5. Dynamic nature of ST segment elevation. (*A*) Prehospital tracing of a patient with left hand weakness and numbness. There is high STE in V1–V4 with upwardly concave ST segments, but also STE in lead aVL with reciprocal depression in inferior leads. (*B*) First tracing in the ED, leads V1–V6 only. STE has resolved spontaneously. The only abnormality is depressed ST segment takeoff in V2 and V3 (limb leads were normal). Moments later, the ST segments re-elevated and the patient rapidly went into cardiogenic shock; he died before the LAD occlusion could be opened.

III) [63]. One should always assess the ST segment deviation, however, within the larger context of overall ECG morphology and clinical presentation. Minimal STE may well be the result of coronary occlusion; conversely, STE exceeding criteria may be the patient's baseline.

With prolonged ischemia, the prominent T waves remain as STE develops. The ST segment evolves from an upwardly concave morphology to one that is straight and then convex (Fig. 6; and see Fig. 4). A concave ST morphology may persist but is more common in nonpathologic states. In anterior AMI, an upwardly concave waveform in V2–V5 is common (Fig. 7; and see Figs. 2 and 5) [64], but upwardly convex morphology is more specific for STEMI and is associated with greater infarct size and morbidity [65]. Coronary occlusion is often transient or dynamic with cyclic reperfusion and reocclusion (see Fig. 5) [66]. Indeed, transient STE caused by spontaneous reperfusion occurs in approximately 20% of STEMI, especially after aspirin therapy [67]. Occlusion may be associated with minimal STE, and if morphology is concave upward, the diagnosis may be missed—but should be suspected if the T wave towers over the R wave or over a Q wave (Fig. 8).

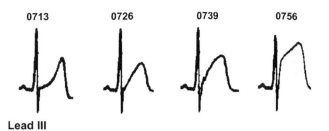

Lead III

Fig. 6. Evolution of ST segment elevation. These single QRS complexes demonstrate the evolution of the ST segment from normal concave upward (0713) to straight (0726) to convex (0739) to still more ST segment elevation, confirming STEMI. *Reprinted with permission from* Chan TC, Brady WJ, Harrigan RA, et al. ECG in emergency medicine and acute care. Elsevier; 2005.

Because of cyclic reperfusion and reocclusion, symptoms may be prolonged in the absence of any significant irreversible infarction; the ECG itself is a better predictor of salvageable myocardium than is symptom duration. In the presence of high STE and high upright T waves, prolonged persistent occlusion with irreversible myocardial damage is unlikely, even with prolonged symptoms [45,47,48].

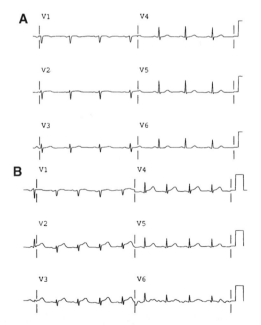

Fig. 7. Subtle ST segment elevation. (*A*) Leads V1–V6 only. Patient with chest pain; ECG shows low voltage only. (*B*) Leads V1–V6 only. Fifty-two minutes later the ECG shows subtle STE in V2–V4, but the STE is more than 50% the amplitude of the QRS complex. She underwent immediate percutaneous coronary intervention for a LAD occlusion.

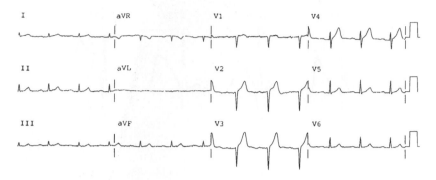

Fig. 8. Unusually large T wave with subtle ST segment elevation. This tracing from a 91-year-old patient with LAD occlusion manifesting as tall T waves that tower over a tiny R wave (V3) and Q wave (V2). This was misinterpreted as early repolarization, which should have well developed R waves and is unusual in elderly patients. The computer did not detect this AMI.

Under the best of circumstances, the ECG has a sensitivity of 56% and specificity of 94% for all AMI as diagnosed by CK-MB [68], but studies vary [12–14]. Even STEMI often is not obvious, and ECG computer algorithms are especially insensitive for this diagnosis (Figs. 8–13) [53,54,69]. Nevertheless, if such algorithms incorporate clinical data, they may increase the percentage of patients who appropriately receive reperfusion therapy [70].

The ECGs with the greatest ST deviation typically result in the shortest time to treatment [71]. Factors such as myocardial mass, distance between the electrodes and the ischemic zone, opposing reciprocal voltage, and especially QRS complex amplitude, may affect the magnitude of STE, so that subtle STE (ie, elevation <2 mm in V1–V3, or ≤1 mm in other leads) may represent persistent coronary occlusion and may be missed easily.

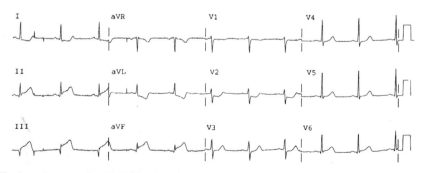

Fig. 9. Inferoposterior STEMI completely missed by the computer. There is a QR wave in lead III very soon after occlusion. There is the obligatory reciprocal ST depression in aVL, and reciprocal STD in V2 and V3 diagnostic of posterior STEMI. STE in lead III is >STE in lead II; there is significant STD in lead I: thus it is an right coronary artery (RCA) occlusion (with posterior branches). Reprinted with permission from: Chan TC, et al. (Eds.), ECG in Emergency Medicine and Acute Care.

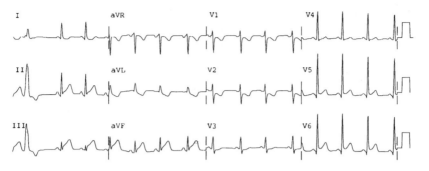

Fig. 10. Inferoposterolateral STEMI completely missed by the computer. There is the obligatory reciprocal ST segment depression in lead aVL, and also reciprocal depression in leads V2 and V3 diagnostic posterior STEMI. Predictors of infarct-related artery are: STE in lead III >STE in lead II (favoring RCA), STD in lead I is minimal (favoring the left circumflex (LCX)), and STE in leads V5 and V6 (favoring LCX); angiography showed LCX occlusion.

Such cases may be difficult to recognize or difficult to differentiate from other etiologies, or both. In the presence of a small QRS, STE may be minimal; amplitude ratios are more accurate than absolute amplitudes [72]. When deciding if any anterior ST elevation is due to left anterior descending coronary artery occlusion vs. due to normal variant, the height of the R wave appears to be most important, with a mean R wave <5 mm in V2-V4 highly suggestive of STEMI [73]. STEMI is defined by STE of at least 1 mm; however, as expertise in ECG interpretation is improving in this era of angiographic correlation, many coronary occlusions manifesting lesser STE, or in only one lead, or simply hyperacute T waves, are being detected and treated with emergent PCI (see Figs. 7 and 11–13). Change from previous ECGs, changes over minutes to hours (see Fig. 7), the presence or absence of reciprocal STD, or presence of upward convexity, may help make the diagnosis. Circumflex or first diagonal occlusion may present with minimal or no STE [74–76] despite large myocardial risk area [77,78], because the lateral wall is more electrocardiographically silent.

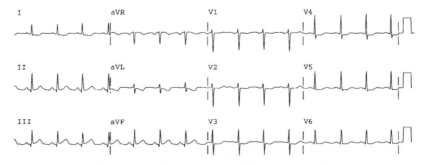

Fig. 11. RCA occlusion manifesting minimal ST deviation, also missed by the computer. There is STE in leads II, III, and aVF with reciprocal depression in leads I, aVL, and leads V2–V5, but all <1 mm.

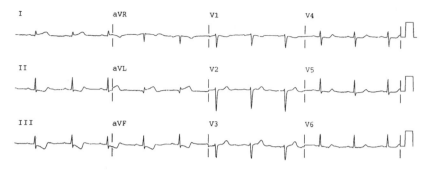

Fig. 12. Obtuse marginal occlusion, also missed by the computer. Reciprocal STD in leads II, III, and aVF is the most visible sign of STEMI. STE is 0.5 mm in leads I and aVL, but in the presence of a low voltage QRS complex. Also, there are nondiagnostic ST segment/T wave changes in leads V4–V6.

Prognostic features of ST segment elevation

The following ECG features of STEMI, in decreasing order of importance, are associated with larger MI, higher mortality, and greater benefit from reperfusion therapy, and may help in determining the benefit/risk ratio of particularly risky (relatively contraindicated) therapies. Though the correlations are real, there remains wide individual variation such that some patients without these features may have a large AMI [79]: (1) anterior location, compared with inferior or lateral [80–84]; (2) total ST deviation or the absolute sum of STE and STD [50,85]; (3) ST score (the sum of all STE) greater than 1.2 mV (12 mm) (these last two features each take into account the prognostic effects of greater height of ST segments and greater number of leads involved) [83]; and (4) distortion of the terminal portion of

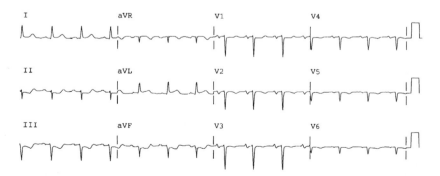

Fig. 13. First diagonal occlusion, also missed by the computer. Reciprocal STD in leads II, III, and aVF is the most visible sign of STEMI. There is left anterior fascicular block, but this does not obscure the diagnosis. STE is 0.5 mm in leads I and aVL, but large compared with a low voltage QRS complex. There is nondiagnostic T-wave inversion in leads V2–V6. Moments later this patient suffered a cardiac arrest. PCI was successful after resuscitation.

the QRS (loss of S-wave in leads with RS configuration, or J point $\geq 50\%$ the height of the R wave) [86] (see Fig. 1).

ST segment depression

Primary STD (Fig. 14)—if not caused by posterior STEMI or reciprocal changes to STE—is an ECG sign of subendocardial ischemia, and in the context of ACS, indicates UA/NSTEMI. STD of even 0.5 mm from baseline is associated with increased mortality, but it is particularly significant when ≥ 1 mm (0.10 mV) in two or more contiguous leads [87]. This adverse prognostic association is independent of elevated troponin [88]. Although STD, especially upsloping STD, may be baseline and stable, the STD associated with UA/NSTEMI is transient and dynamic. Its morphology is usually flat or downsloping. Concurrent T-wave inversion may or may not be present. STD may be induced by exercise in the presence of stable coronary stenosis. Just as with STE, the proportionality or lead strength of STD is important: 1 mm of STD following a <10 mm R wave is more specific for ischemia but less *sensitive* than is 1 mm of STD following a >20 mm R wave [89–92].

STD >2 mm and present in three or more leads is associated with a high probability of elevated CK-MB and near universal elevation of troponin. In the absence of PCI, such STD is associated with a 30-day mortality of up to 35% and a 4-year mortality of 47% [93], whether or not there is complete coronary occlusion. Lesser degrees of STD (in the absence of PCI) are associated with 30-day mortality rates from 10%–26% [85,94] and also with a high incidence of left main or three-vessel disease [95]. Primary STD, with the exception of that which represents posterior STEMI or that which is reciprocal to other STE, is not an indication for thrombolytic therapy [96–98]. In the pre-interventional era, patients who had STD and AMI (by

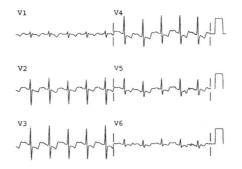

Fig. 14. ST segment depression. Leads V1–V6 only. Flat STD of LAD subendocardial ischemia is likely when STD reaches from leads V2–V6 and is transient. Thrombolytic therapy thus is not indicated. Furthermore, as in most UA/NSTEMI, the STD resolved quickly with medical therapy.

CK-MB) had a higher mortality than those with STE who were eligible for thrombolytics (STEMI) and received them [94,99]. STD (even as little as 0.5 mm) [87,95], independently of and in addition to elevated troponin, is a strong predictor of adverse outcome and is one of the best indicators of benefit from early (within 48 hours) PCI, in addition to intensive medical therapy [1,95]. Persistent STD in the setting of persistent angina despite maximal medical therapy is an indication for urgent angiography with possible percutaneous coronary intervention, but not for thrombolytic therapy.

Reciprocal STD is the electrical mirroring phenomenon observed on the ventricular wall opposite transmural injury (see Figs. 4, 5, 9, and 10). This simultaneous STD improves the specificity for STEMI in the anatomic territory of the STE, but true reciprocal STD does not reflect ischemia in the territory of the STD. Hence, in the reciprocal territory, there will be no associated wall motion abnormality on echocardiogram or myocardial perfusion defect with nuclear imaging. Because a significant number of STEMIs do not develop reciprocal STD, absence of reciprocal ST depression does not rule out STEMI [16,100–104]. In the presence of abnormal conduction (eg, left ventricular hypertrophy [LVH], bundle branch block [BBB], or intraventricular conduction delay [IVCD]), STD may be secondary to this abnormal QRS complex, and, if so, it does not contribute substantially to the diagnosis [104].

Three situations frequently are called reciprocal; only the first represents true reciprocity or mirroring of STE present on the 12-lead: (1) true reciprocity of the leads with STE (eg, in inferior AMI, reciprocal STD in lead aVL, which is 150° opposite from lead III [see Fig. 9]); (2) posterior STEMI (ie, ST depression in leads V1–V4, with or without STE in leads V5 and V6 or leads II, III, and aVF), (Fig. 15; see Figs. 9 and 10). In this case, the STD is truly reciprocal, but only to what *would be* STE on posterior leads, not to inferior or lateral STE; (3) simultaneous UA/NSTEMI of another coronary distribution (not in any way reciprocal).

Anterior AMI manifests reciprocal STD in at least one of leads II, III, and aVF in 40%–70% of cases; this STD correlates strongly with a proximal left anterior descending (LAD) occlusion (see Figs. 4 and 5) [105–108]. In the presence of inferior AMI, reciprocal STD usually is present in leads I and aVL, and often in the precordial leads, especially V1–V3 (56% of cases) [109]. Reciprocal STD is associated with a higher mortality [85], but also with greater benefit from thrombolytics [50]. This is especially true of precordial STD in inferior AMI [109]. In some cases, reciprocal STD is the most visible sign of STEMI (see Figs. 4, 12, and 13) [34,110].

T-wave inversion

In the presence of normal conduction, the normal T-wave axis is toward the apex of the heart and is close to the QRS axis: the T wave is usually upright in the left-sided leads I, II, and V3–V6; inverted in lead aVR; and

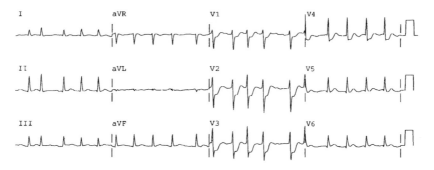

Fig. 15. Acute posterior wall MI. There is no ST segment elevation on this ECG, yet this patient is a candidate for thrombolytics. The marked ST segment depression in leads V1–V4 was a reciprocal view of a posterior wall STEMI. Angiography revealed an occluded second obtuse marginal artery.

variable in leads III, aVL, aVF, and V1, with rare normal inversion in V2. When abnormally inverted, if in the presence of symptoms suggesting ACS, such T waves should be assumed to be a manifestation of ischemia, although there are many nonischemic etiologies of T-wave inversion. Isolated or minimally inverted nondynamic T waves (<1 mm) may be caused by ACS but have not been shown to be associated with adverse outcomes compared with patients who have ACS and a normal ECG [95]; however, T-wave inversion caused by ACS that is >1 mm or in ≥2 leads is associated a higher risk of complications, especially if of Wellens pattern [111,112].

T-wave inversion caused by ACS may be transient (reversible) and may be without significant ST segment shift, indicating transient ischemia. In such a case there is usually no myocardial damage, as measured by troponin, and it is diagnosed as UA.

In general, sustained and evolving regional T-wave inversion suggests either (1) spontaneous reperfusion (of the infarct artery or through collaterals) (Fig. 16), or (2), in the presence of QS waves, prolonged occlusion (Fig. 17). After prolonged, non-reperfused coronary occlusion, as regional ST segments resolve toward the isoelectric level, T waves invert in the same region, but not deeply (up to 3 mm) [113]. Shallow T-wave inversions in the presence of deep QS waves recorded at patient presentation usually represent prolonged persistent occlusion, with (nearly) completed infarction [113]. Even with ongoing STE, it may be too late for thrombolytic therapy.

With reperfusion, whether spontaneous or as a result of therapy or caused by collateral flow, there is often regional terminal T-wave inversion [114,115]. This terminal inversion is identical to Wellens pattern A [34,111] and the cove-plane T [114,115]. The ST segments may retain some elevation, but the T waves invert, resulting in a biphasic appearance (Fig. 18A).

As time progresses after reperfusion, the ST segments recover to near the isoelectric level, are upwardly convex, and the inversion is more symmetric

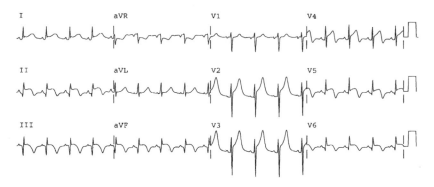

Fig. 16. Occlusion with reperfusion of a wraparound RCA, similar to a wraparound LAD (anterior and inferior AMI). Such widespread STE (inferior, anterior, lateral) with no reciprocal STD (it is absent in lead aVL because of lateral AMI) if the T waves are still upright, frequently is misdiagnosed as pericarditis. Inferior and lateral cove-plane (inverted) T waves clinch the diagnosis of AMI and signify reperfusion of these regions. Angiography confirmed inferior and lateral reperfusion by way of collaterals, but persistent ischemia to the anterior wall.

and deep (>3 mm) [113]. This is identical to Wellens pattern B [34,111] or the coronary T or Pardee T [116,117] (Fig. 18B and 19).

In both types of Wellens T-wave inversions, the R wave is preserved because reperfusion occurs before irreversible necrosis; both are believed to be a result of ischemia surrounding the infarct zone. If the T-wave inversion is persistent, there is nearly always some minimal troponin elevation, and this pattern frequently is termed non-Q wave MI. If no STE was recorded, this is appropriately termed NSTEMI, though frequently transient STE would have been present had an ECG been obtained at the appropriate moment.

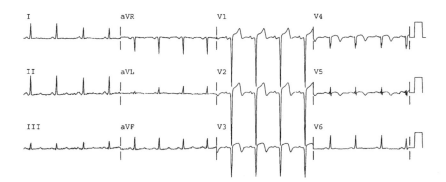

Fig. 17. Anterior STE with QS waves and terminal T-wave inversion. This is diagnostic of STE-MI, but QS waves suggest prolonged occlusion and deep T-wave inversion suggests (late) spontaneous reperfusion. Indeed, this 37-year-old patient's symptoms had been constant for 32 hours. CK was 5615 IU/L. The LAD, however, was persistently occluded at angiography. *Reprinted with permission from* Smith SW, Zvosec DL, Sharkey SW, Henry TD. The ECG in acute MI: an evidence-based manual of reperfusion therapy. Fig. 33-8. 1st edition. Philadelphia: Lippincott, Williams, and Wilkins: 2002. p. 358.

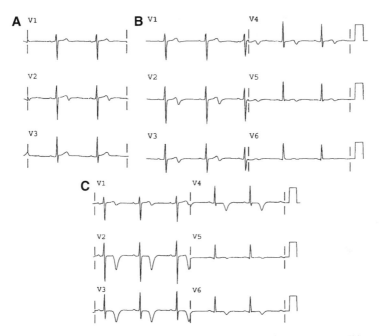

Fig. 18. Wellens syndrome. (*A*) Wellens syndrome, pattern A (leads V1–V3 only). This patient's chest pain had resolved recently and he now has subtle biphasic terminal T-wave inversion in lead V2; although the QT interval is short, suggesting benign T-wave inversion, but this would be unusual in lead V2 only. (*B*) Wellens syndrome, pattern A (leads V1–V6 only): the same patient 2 hours later. The ECG now has biphasic terminal T-wave inversion in V2–V5. The QTc interval is 0.45 sec, more typical of Wellens syndrome. This also helps to differentiate from benign T-wave inversion (QTc <0.40–0.425 sec). Troponin but not CK-MB was minimally elevated and there was a very tight LAD stenosis at angiography. (*C*) Wellens pattern B (leads V1–V6 only). The same patient 9 hours later. The T waves are now monophasic, inverted, and deep.

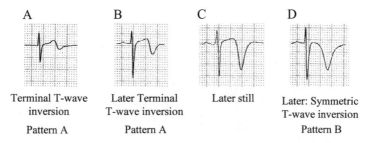

A	B	C	D
Terminal T-wave inversion	Later Terminal T-wave inversion	Later still	Later: Symmetric T-wave inversion
Pattern A	Pattern A		Pattern B

Fig. 19. Evolution of T-wave inversion (*A–D*) after coronary reperfusion in STEMI reperfusion and in Wellens syndrome (NSTEMI). *Reprinted with permission from* Smith SW, Zvosec DL, Sharkey SW, Henry TD. The ECG in acute MI: an evidence-based manual of reperfusion therapy. 1st edition. Philadelphia: Lippincott, Williams, and Wilkins: 2002. p. 358.

Wellens syndrome (see Fig. 18*A*,*B*) refers to angina with T-wave inversion in the LAD distribution, particularly V2–V4, in the presence of persistent R waves [34,111,118,119] and critical stenosis of the LAD [111,112]. At initial presentation, patients have normal or slightly elevated CK-MB and elevated troponin. The ECG pattern is present in a pain-free state. Wellens' group noted, however, that without angioplasty, 75% of these patients developed an anterior wall AMI, usually within a matter of days, despite relief of symptoms with medical management. Identical T-wave morphology is recorded after approximately 60% of cases of successful reperfusion therapy for anterior STEMI [114,115], suggesting that Wellens syndrome is a clinical condition created by spontaneous reperfusion of a previously occluded critical stenosis. Similar patterns also occur in other coronary distributions, eg, inferior, lateral, or both (see Fig. 16), but the syndrome was described originally in the LAD. Wellens syndrome is to be distinguished from benign T-wave inversion by (1) longer QT interval (>425 ms as opposed to <400–425 ms) and (2) location V2–V4 (as opposed to V3–V5).

In the presence of prior T-wave inversion, reocclusion of the coronary artery manifests as ST segment re-elevation and normalization of terminal T-wave inversion, called T-wave pseudonormalization because the T wave flips upright (Fig. 20). With upright T waves, pseudonormalization should not be assumed if the previous ECG showing T-wave inversion was recorded more than 1 month earlier.

T-wave inversions with no STE are never an indication for thrombolytics. With symptoms of ACS, they represent UA/NSTEMI. Even in the presence

Reocclusion

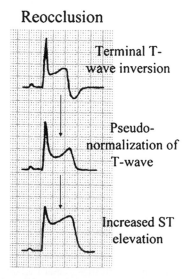

Terminal T-wave inversion

Pseudo-normalization of T-wave

Increased ST elevation

Fig. 20. Pseudonormalization of inverted T waves. *Reprinted with permission from* Smith SW, Zvosec DL, Sharkey SW, Henry TD. The ECG in acute MI: an evidence-based manual of reperfusion therapy. 1st edition. Philadelphia: Lippincott, Williams, and Wilkins: 2002. p. 358.

of persistent STE, they usually indicate spontaneous reperfusion or collateral flow, or, if new Q waves are present, a prolonged occlusion; thrombolytics should be given only if ongoing chest pain suggests persistent occlusion and serial ECGs fail to show resolution of STE (see Fig. 16).

Q waves

Before the thrombolytic era, MI was classified based on its clinical pathology: either as Q wave or non-Q wave MI, or as transmural versus subendocardial MI [120]. These terms later were discovered to be clinically and pathologically unrelated. Q waves correlate with the volume of infarcted myocardium, rather than the transmural extent of MI [121]. The Q wave/non-Q wave distinction remains useful, because Q waves are associated with a lower ejection fraction and a larger MI [121–125]. Most patients with non-reperfused STEMI ultimately develop Q waves, whereas a minority do not [126]; in any case, they often appear after the important initial diagnostic and therapeutic interventions have occurred. Hence, AMI is now classified as STEMI or NSTEMI.

A normal Q wave representing the rapid depolarization of the thin septal wall between the two ventricles may be found in most leads (Box 1). This initial negative deflection of the QRS complex is of short duration and of low amplitude. Pathologic Q waves, often a consequence of MI, are generally wider and deeper than normal Q waves. Following MI with significant

---

Box 1. Abnormal Q waves

- Lead V2: any Q wave
- Lead V3: almost any Q wave
- Lead V4: >1 mm deep *or* at least 0.02 sec *or* larger than the Q wave in lead V5
- Any Q wave ≥0.03 sec (30 ms, 0.75 mm), except in leads III, aVR, or V1 (see below)
- Lead aVL: Q wave >0.04 sec or >50% of the amplitude of the QRS in the presence of an upright p-wave
- Lead III: Q wave ≥0.04 sec. A Q wave of depth >25% of R wave height is often quoted as diagnostic, but width is more important than depth
- Leads III, aVR, V1: normal subjects may have nonpathologic wide and deep Q waves

---

Adapted with permission from Smith SW, Zvosec DL, Sharkey SW, Henry TD. The ECG in acute MI: an evidence-based manual of reperfusion therapy. 1st edition. Philadelphia: Lippincott, Williams, and Wilkins: 2002. p. 358.

loss of myocardium, electrically inactive tissue fails to produce an R wave in the overlying leads; depolarization of the opposite wall in the opposite direction then gets recorded negatively (Q wave). A QR wave denotes a Q wave followed by a substantial R wave (see Fig. 16, inferior leads); a Qr wave denotes a Q wave followed by a very small R wave (see Fig. 9, lead III); a qR wave denotes a small Q wave preceding a large R wave (see Fig. 16, lateral leads); and a QS wave denotes a single negative deflection without any R wave (see Fig. 17).

There are several Q wave equivalents seen in the precordial leads. These include (1) R wave diminution—or poor R wave progression; (2) reverse R wave progression, in which R waves increase then decrease in amplitude across the precordial leads (although this must be distinguished from precordial electrode misconnection); and (3) tall R waves in leads V1 and V2, representing "Q waves" of posterior infarction.

Because Q waves commonly are considered markers of irreversible infarction, reperfusion therapy often is denied to patients whose ECGs already manifest Q waves. By 60 minutes after LAD occlusion, however, QR waves, but usually not QS waves, occur in the right precordial leads in 50% of patients, and they frequently disappear after reperfusion [127]. These QR waves are caused by ischemia of the conducting system and not irreversible infarction [29]. Although patients who have high ST segments and absence of Q waves have the greatest benefit from thrombolytic therapy, those who have high ST segment elevation and QR waves also receive significant benefit (see Figs. 9 and 16) [29,30]. Q waves signifying necrosis should be developed completely within 8–12 hours of onset of persistent occlusion [29,30], although at least 10% of patients do not develop them for up to 2 weeks [128]. In most patients, these Q waves persist indefinitely, but in up to 30% of AMI that receives no reperfusion therapy, the Q waves eventually disappear [129]. In contrast, when patients who have Q waves receive early thrombolytic therapy, the Q waves disappear within a few days to weeks [30,130].

Significance of pathologic Q waves for reperfusion therapy in acute coronary syndromes

When the significance of STE is uncertain, the presence of a pathologic QR wave in that lead increases the probability that the STE is caused by AMI (not pseudoinfarction) and is amenable to immediate reperfusion. Pathologic QR waves with or without acute ST segment/T-wave changes increase the likelihood of ACS, because it is strong evidence of the presence of coronary artery disease (CAD). Because pathologic QR waves may be present very early in AMI, and because they are associated with benefit from thrombolytic therapy [29], they should not in any way dissuade from reperfusion therapy. A QS pattern caused by MI represents lack of any R wave depolarization of normal tissue, and thus usually indicates significant irreversible myocardial loss (see Fig. 17). QS waves in leads V1–V3, which may occur with STE, also may be caused by LBBB, left ventricular hypertrophy (LVH), cor pulmonale, or cardiomyopathy. If STE without *deep* T-wave inversion exists in the presence of a QS wave, LV aneurysm also should be considered.

Reperfusion and reocclusion

Together with angiographic evidence of microvascular perfusion, resolution of STE is the best predictor of outcome from STEMI [34,131]. On continuous ST segment monitoring after reperfusion therapy, a recovery of the ST segment to <50% of its maximal height by 60 minutes is associated strongly with TIMI-3 reperfusion, and even more strongly associated with good microvascular perfusion [132].

A less sensitive but highly specific predictor of reperfusion is terminal T-wave inversion identical to that of Wellens T waves (see Figs. 16, 18, and 19) [114,115]. In patients who have STEMI, the presence of negative T waves very early after presentation or very soon after therapy is associated with a good prognosis [48]. Negative T waves at discharge of patients who have anterior STEMI is correlated strongly with ST recovery to baseline and TIMI-3 flow [133]. Whether reperfusion is spontaneous or therapy-induced, reocclusion can be detected by re-elevation of ST segments or by pseudonormalization of inverted T waves within hours, days, or weeks of the index AMI (Fig. 20). It may be confused with postinfarction regional pericarditis. T-wave normalization beyond 1 month is expected without reocclusion and is not necessarily pseudonormalization.

Regional issues in acute coronary syndrome

Anterior myocardial infarction

Anatomy

See Table 1 for correlations between coronary occlusion and location of STEMI, and Fig. 21 for coronary anatomy.

The left main coronary artery supplies the LAD artery and the left circumflex (LCX) artery. Persistent occlusion of the left main usually leads to cardiogenic shock and death. The LAD supplies the anterior wall, with branches supplying the anterolateral wall (diagonal arteries) and most of the septum (septal arteries); it may extend distally around the apex to the inferior wall ("wrap-around" LAD) (see Fig. 16). The first septal branch (S1) usually originates from the LAD proximal to the first diagonal branch (D1); but in some it originates distal to D1. The ramus intermedius may arise at the division of the left main, producing a trifurcation, and is present in one third of subjects [134]. It supplies the anterolateral wall.

Table 1
ST elevation, location of STEMI, and corresponding coronary artery

ST elevation	Coronary artery (see Fig. 21)	AMI location
II, III, aVF (reciprocal ST depression in aVL)	RCA 80% (III >II, STD in I) Dominant circumflex (II>III, no STD in I)	Inferior AMI
II, III, aVF (reciprocal ST depression in aVL) plus V1 Right-sided ECG: V4R	RCA proximal to RV marginal branch	Inferior and RV AMI
II, III, aVF (reciprocal ST depression in aVL) plus ST depression in V1–V4	Dominant RCA (70%) Dominant circumflex (30%)	Inferoposterior AMI
II, III, aVF plus (I, aVL and/or V5, V6)	Dominant circumflex **or** Dominant RCA with lateral branches	Inferolateral AMI
II, III, aVF plus (V5, V6) and/or (I, aVL) and ST depression any of V1–V6	Dominant RCA with lateral branches or circumflex	Inferoposterolateral AMI
V2–V4	Mid LAD, distal to diagonal and septal perforator	Anterior AMI
I, aVL, V5 and/or V6, sometimes minimal; inferior reciprocal STD very common, may be most obvious feature	First diagonal or circumflex or obtuse marginal artery	Lateral AMI
V1–V3, sometimes out to V5, with V1>V2>V3>V4>V5, with or without inferior STE or Qs Also V1R–V6R, especially V4R	Right ventricular marginal (RVM), or by occlusion of RCA proximal to RVM	Right ventricular AMI (pseudoanteroseptal AMI)
V1–V4, often without inferior reciprocal STD	LAD, possibly proximal to first septal perforator but distal to first diagonal	Anteroseptal AMI
V1–V6, I, aVL, 80% with 1 mm STD in II, III, and aVF	Proximal LAD	Anteroseptallateral AMI
STD in V1–V4, with or without lateral or inferior STE	LCX (absence of STE is possible, or lateral only) RCA (inferior STE, +/− lateral)	Posterior AMI

Adapted with permission from Smith SW, Zvosec DL, Sharkey SW, Henry TD. The ECG in acute MI: an evidence-based manual of reperfusion therapy. 1st edition. Philadelphia: Lippincott, Williams, and Wilkins; 2002. p. 358.

There is great variation among patients. Use this for guidelines only.

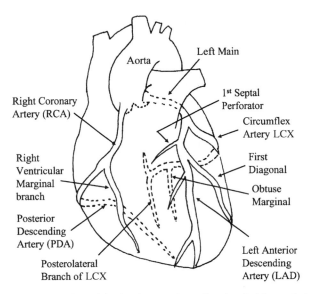

Fig. 21. Coronary anatomy in a right dominant system. *Reprinted with permission from* Smith SW, Zvosec DL, Sharkey SW, Henry TD. The ECG in acute MI: an evidence-based manual of reperfusion therapy. Fig. 4–5. 1st edition. Philadelphia: Lippincott, Williams, and Wilkins: 2002. p. 358.

Mid left anterior descending occlusion (anterior acute myocardial infarction)

STE in V2–V4, sometimes including V1, is the hallmark of occlusion distal to S1 and D1. There is frequently no inferior reciprocal STD (see Fig. 8). In the presence of a wrap-around LAD, there also may be STE in leads II, III and aVF (see Fig. 16).

Proximal left anterior descending occlusion (anterolateral, anteroseptal, anteroseptolateral acute myocardial infarction)
Lateral component. LAD occlusion proximal to D1 manifests as anterolateral AMI (with STE in leads V2–V4, maximal in V2–V3), and STE in lead aVL and occasionally leads I and V5–V6. Inferior reciprocal STD is present in approximately 80% of cases, depending largely on how STD is defined in number of leads and depth of depression [106,107]. These ST depressions are often reciprocal to STE in leads I and aVL, or to high anterobasal STE in V1. Together with STE in V2–V4, STE in aVL >0.5 mm is very sensitive, and >1.0 mm very specific, for occlusion of the LAD proximal to D1 [104]. Echocardiographic studies comparing proximal and distal occlusions show no difference in apical wall motion [135,136] (see Figs. 2 and 5).

Septal component. STE in V1 traditionally indicates occlusion proximal to S1 with involvement of the septum (anteroseptal MI). Using echocardiography, STE in V1, but not VZ, is associated with basal anterior, anteroseptal and septal regional dysfunction [136]. STE in V1 is not very specific, however, unless >2.5 mm [107]. Other predictors of occlusion proximal to S1 are (1) STE in lead aVR, (2) STD in lead III >STE in lead aVL, (3) ST segment depression in V5, and (4) right BBB (RBBB) [107,108].

Lateral and posterior acute myocardial infarction

Anatomy

The left main bifurcates into the LAD and LCX. The lateral wall of the LV is supplied by the LCX and its obtuse marginal (OM) branches and occasionally by D1 from the LAD. When the LCX wraps around to *both* the posterobasal (posterior) and posteroapical (inferior) walls, giving off the posterior descending artery (PDA), it is the dominant vessel, meaning occlusion results in inferior AMI (STE in II, III, and aVF). Branches of a large dominant right coronary artery (RCA) also may supply the posterolateral wall [137]. Occlusion of a nondominant LCX or one of its obtuse marginal branches accounts for most isolated posterior AMIs (lateral AMI may be present, but rarely pronounced).

Lateral acute myocardial infarction

Lateral AMI is a result of occlusion of D1 off the LAD, or of the LCX or its obtuse marginal branches. It may be simultaneous with anterior AMI if the occlusion is in the LAD proximal to D1; it may be simultaneous with posterior AMI in occlusion of the LCX, and with posterior and inferior AMI in occlusion of a *dominant* LCX (see Fig. 10) or dominant RCA. STE is often <1 mm (0.1 mV), especially in aVL, and especially with low QRS voltage (see Figs. 12 and 13). The sensitivity of STE for detection of lateral AMI is low: with LCX occlusion there is (1) STE in inferior or lateral leads in only 36%, (2) STE >2 mm in only 5%, (3) Isolated STD in 30%, (4) some STE or STD in two thirds of cases, and (5) neither STE nor STD in 33% [74–76,138–140]. This contrasts markedly with LAD or RCA occlusion, which manifest STE in 70%–92% of cases [74,75]. Reciprocal STD in inferior leads is often the most pronounced effect of occlusion of D1 or an OM. STD in V5, V6, and aVL also corresponds with disrupted perfusion of D1 or OM1. Lateral AMI caused by LCX or OM occlusion frequently is accompanied by posterior AMI (see later discussion) (see Figs. 12 and 13).

Posterior acute myocardial infarction

From 3.3%–8.5% of all AMIs as diagnosed by CK-MB are posterior AMIs that present without STE on the standard 12-lead ECG, and thus the diagnosis often is missed (see Fig. 15) [34,78,141–144]. These isolated posterior wall AMIs usually present with precordial reciprocal STD, however, often upsloping, in leads V1–V4. STD in V1–V4 may be caused by anterior subendocardial ischemia of the LAD, but this is usually downsloping and transient and extends out to V6 (see Fig. 14). Most individuals have some STE at baseline in V2 and V3 [17], and any amount of STD may represent a large change in ST amplitude (delta ST). As always, comparison with a baseline tracing is helpful.

Posterior leads V7–V9 reveal posterior STE (Fig. 22). Leads V7–V9 are more specific than precordial leads for posterior AMI (84% versus 57%), with similar sensitivity for both (approximately 80%) [145]. If 0.5 mm is used as a cutoff in leads V7–V9, sensitivity is greatly enhanced but with an unknown change in specificity [144]. Placement of V7–V9 should be in the fifth intercostal space (at the same level as V6), with V7 at the posterior axillary line, V8 at the scapular tip, and V9 at the left paraspinal border. Routine use of posterior leads for all patients who have chest pain is unwarranted, because the vast majority are normal [146,147].

Inferior and right ventricular acute myocardial infarction

Anatomy

The RCA is the dominant vessel in 80% of individuals; that is, it gives off the PDA to supply the inferior wall. The LCX is dominant in 20%, in which case the RCA supplies little more than the right ventricle (RV). RCA occlusion is the most common cause of inferior AMI. Occlusion proximal to the RV marginal branch of the RCA results in concurrent RV AMI (Fig. 23). Occlusion of the RCA with a large posterolateral branch leads to inferolateral, inferoposterior (see Fig. 9), or inferoposterolateral AMI. Occlusion of the LCX in a left-dominant heart manifests as an inferoposterolateral AMI (see Fig. 10). Inferior AMI produces STE in II, III, and aVF. There is almost always reciprocal STD in lead aVL. On occasion, lateral AMI hides

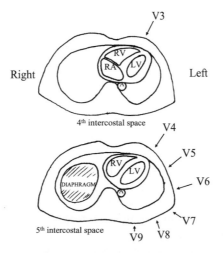

Fig. 22. Placement of posterior electrodes (V7, V8, and V9) for detection of posterior MI. *Reprinted with permission from* Smith SW, Zvosec DL, Sharkey SW, Henry TD. The ECG in acute MI: an evidence-based manual of reperfusion therapy. 1st edition. Philadelphia: Lippincott, Williams, and Wilkins: 2002. p. 358.

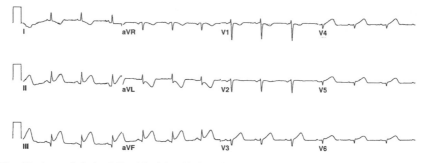

Fig. 23. Acute inferior MI with right-sided leads reflecting RV involvement. The limb leads demonstrate STE in the inferior leads (lead III>lead II), together with reciprocal STD in lead aVL>lead I—all suggesting RCA occlusion. The precordial leads are actually leads V1R–V6R, or right-sided leads. The STE in leads V3R–V6R indicate RV infarction.

this, and there is usually STE in V5 or V6; however, if STD in aVL is not present, the diagnosis of inferior AMI must be questioned (see Fig. 16).

Determining the culprit vessel may be important: RCA occlusion, if proximal, leads to RV AMI and may result in hypotension, which responds well to fluids and can be exacerbated greatly by nitrates.

LCX (versus RCA) occlusion is strongly predicted by (1) greater STE in lead II than in lead III, and by (2) the absence of reciprocal STD in lead I [148,149], but also by (3) isoelectric or elevated ST segment in lead I or aVL [150], (4) an abnormally tall R wave in lead V1 [74], or (4) STE in lateral precordial leads V5 and V6 [150]. Additionally, ECG findings of RV AMI suggest RCA occlusion (see later discussion).

RCA occlusion is strongly predicted by (1) STE in lead III >II [149], (2) STD in lead I or aVL with deviation in lead aVL >lead I [150,151], (3) STE in V1, V4R, or both, and (4) STE in V1–V4, a sign of concomitant RV involvement (Fig. 24) [152].

In inferior AMI, simultaneous STD in leads V1–V4 reflects concurrent posterior wall injury (it infrequently reflects anterior wall subendocardial ischemia) and a larger amount of myocardium at risk, higher mortality, and greater benefit from reperfusion; however, this finding does not discriminate between LCX or RCA occlusions [105,109,150,153,154] (see Figs. 9 and 10).

Inferior AMI is sometimes associated with conduction defects at the AV node, including first degree AV block, Mobitz type I (but not type II) or Wenkebach-type AV block, and complete heart block. With complete block, there is usually a stable junctional rhythm with narrow QRS and pulse rate greater than 40 beats per minute (BPM). It is typically transient, and does not require permanent pacing. This type of AV block contrasts sharply to that associated with an extensive anterior AMI. In this infrequent condition the conduction block occurs distal to the AV node, and is associated with Mobitz type II AV block, bifasicular block, or complete heart block. Here, the complete block manifests as a wide junctional or ventricular escape rhythm less

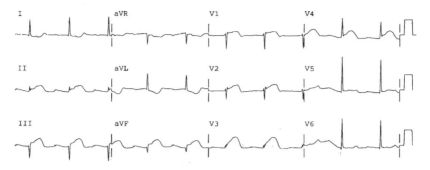

Fig. 24. Unusual presentation of proximal RCA occlusion. Inferior STE with reciprocal STD in leads I and aVL is suspicious for RCA occlusion. STE in lead V1 is typical for RV AMI and normally would confirm the RCA as the infarct artery. There is in addition, however, widespread STE that is unusual for simultaneous LAD occlusion or for pseudo-anteroseptal (RV) AMI; the latter usually have maximal STE in V1 and V2, not V3. The right-sided ECG (not shown) had STE in leads V3R–V6R also.

than 40 BPM. These patients often present or soon develop cardiogenic shock and have significant mortality regardless of temporary pacing.

Right ventricular acute myocardial infarction

Right ventricular acute myocardial infarction (RV AMI) should be suspected when there is acute (or old) inferior MI caused by RCA occlusion (see previous discussion), especially if there is STE in V1 or clinical hypotension. RV AMI is seen in practice exclusively with proximal RCA occlusion or branch occlusion of an RV marginal artery. RV AMI has high short-term morbidity and mortality, especially without reperfusion [155–157], but patients who survive beyond 10 days have a good prognosis [158]. RV AMI

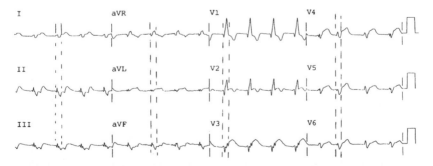

Fig. 25. RBBB with AMI from proximal LAD occlusion. In the presence of RBBB, STE (leads V2–V6, I, and aVL) and reciprocal STD (leads II, III, and aVF) are seen clearly as long as the end of the QRS complex is properly located. Note that in lead V1, although the T wave is appropriately discordant for RBBB, the ST segment is inappropriately normal; it would be expected to be depressed in nonischemic RBBB.

Box 2. Sgarbossa criteria for diagnosis of STEMI in the presence of LBBB

Concordant ST segment elevation ≥1 mm in one or more leads, which means ST segment elevation in leads in which the QRS complex is predominantly positive (V5, V6, I, aVL, or II)
Concordant ST segment depression ≥1 mm in one or more leads (ie, ST segment depression in leads in which QRS complex is predominantly negative [V1, V2, V3]); this is 90% specific for AMI caused by posterior injury
Discordant ST segment elevation ≥5 mm that is excessive (out of proportion) to the depth of the preceding S wave seems to be approximately 90% specific for AMI

---

is often associated with conduction defects at the AV node, including complete heart block.

Isolated RV AMI presents with STE in V1–V3, and it may mimic LAD occlusion (pseudo-anteroseptal AMI), except that the STE usually peaks in V1 or V2 and declines progressively as far as V5, whereas in LAD occlusion, STE peaks in V2 and V3 [152]. Large RV AMI may seem to be an anterior MI (of the LV) even in the presence of inferior STE (Fig. 24). Such extensive and profound STE is especially true in the presence of RV hypertrophy [34,159].

When RCA occlusion is suspected, record a right-sided ECG in which lead V1 becomes lead V2R, lead V2 becomes lead V1R, and leads V3R–

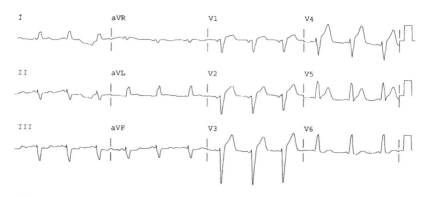

Fig. 26. STEMI in the presence of LBBB. The previous ECG (not shown) had LBBB with typical discordant ST segments and T waves. There is now concordant STE and upright T waves in leads I, aVL, V5, and V6. There is concordant reciprocal STD in the inferior leads II, III, and aVF. LAD occlusion was opened with percutaneous coronary intervention *Reprinted with permission from* Chan TC, Brady WJ, Harrigan RA, et al. ECG in emergency medicine and acute care. Fig. 26-B. Elsevier; 2005.

V6R are placed across the right chest in mirror image to their left precordial counterparts (ie, V3–V6). Q waves across the right-sided ECG are normal. Absence of STE in leads V2R–V7R nearly rules out RV AMI. One millimeter of STE in lead V4R alone has a sensitivity and predictive accuracy for RV infarction of 93% [155,160]. STE up to 0.6 mm in V4R may be normal; however, in the context of inferior AMI, STE >0.5 mm should be interpreted as RV AMI (see Fig. 23) [161,162].

Right and left bundle branch block

AMI with associated RBBB or LBBB is greatly under treated with reperfusion therapy [163]. BBB is associated with a high mortality (8.7%) compared with normal conduction (3.5%), especially if persistent (20%) versus transient (5.6%). Mortality with persistent LBBB was 36% versus 12% for RBBB; both were associated with LAD occlusion in approximately 50% of cases [164].

In RBBB, the ST segment is, by general consensus and by electrophysiologic theory, as reliable as it is in normal conduction. Assessment of ST segment amplitude (ie, of STE), however, may be hindered by difficulty in determining where the QRS complex ends and the ST segment begins. To do so, examine other leads to find the true QRS complex duration, and then compare that millisecond measurement within the lead in question. The J point is then at the end of this measured QRS. The T wave in RBBB usually is inverted in leads with an rSR' (right precordial leads), often with up to 1 mm of STD, especially in lead V2. This should not be mistaken for primary STD. Because of this STD secondary to RBBB, minimal STE may represent a large delta ST (Fig. 25); comparison with a previous ECG may be invaluable. Finally, RBBB in the presence of LV aneurysm may present with a QR wave and STE that mimics acute MI.

The ST segment/T-wave complex in uncomplicated LBBB is opposite in direction (discordant) to most of the QRS complex. To the uninitiated, this normal STE may mimic AMI. Furthermore, LBBB also has a reputation for hiding AMI. There is some electrophysiologic rationale for this. The clinical data, however, may have suffered at the hands of the following faulty logic [165]: only 40%–50% of AMI (by CK-MB) in the presence of LBBB have diagnostic criteria as defined by Sgarbossa and colleagues (Box 2) [165–170]. What may be forgotten is that this is also true of normal conduction: approximately 45% of AMI (by CK-MB) in normal conduction manifests diagnostic STE [12–14]. It seems that the Sgarbossa criteria have similar sensitivity and specificity for AMI (as does STE in normal conduction) and are as sensitive and specific for detection of ongoing epicardial coronary occlusion that requires emergent reperfusion therapy (ie, STEMI). Nevertheless, until there are more data, it is prudent to also treat patients who have high suspicion of AMI and *new* LBBB with reperfusion therapy, even in the absence of Sgarbossa criteria. Additionally, comparison with a previous ECG and serial ECGs are useful for identifying coronary occlusion in the presence of LBBB [34,168,171,172] (Fig. 26).

References

[1] Cannon CP, Weintraub WS, Demopoulos LA, et al. Comparison of early invasive and conservative strategies in patients with unstable coronary syndromes treated with the glycoprotein IIb/IIIa inhibitor tirofiban. (TACTICS)-TIMI 18. N Engl J Med 2001; 344:1879–87.

[2] Eagle KA, Goodman SG, Avezum A, et al. Practice variation and missed opportunities for reperfusion in ST segment-elevation myocardial infarction: findings from the Global Registry of Acute Coronary Events (GRACE). Lancet 2002;359:373–7.

[3] Barron HV, Bowlby LJ, Breen T, et al. Use of reperfusion therapy for acute myocardial infarction in the United States: data from the National Registry of Myocardial Infarction 2. Circulation 1997;97:1150–6.

[4] Hirvonen TP, Halinen MO, Kala RA, et al. Delays in thrombolytic therapy for acute myocardial infarction in Finland. Results of a national thrombolytic therapy delay study. Finnish Hospitals' Thrombolysis Survey Group. Eur Heart J 1998;19:885–92.

[5] Krumholz HM, Murillo JE, Chen J, et al. Thrombolytic therapy for eligible elderly patients with acute myocardial infarction. JAMA 1997;277:1683–8.

[6] Shlipak MG, Go AS, Frederick PD. Treatment and outcomes of left bundle-branch block patients with myocardial infarction who present without chest pain. J Am Coll Cardiol 2000;36:706–12.

[7] Lee TH, Rouan GW, Weisberg MC, et al. Clinical characteristics and natural history of patients with acute myocardial infarction sent home from the emergency room. Am J Cardiol 1987;60:219–24.

[8] McCarthy BD, Beshansky JR, D'Agostino RB, et al. Missed diagnosis of acute myocardial infarction in the emergency department: results from a multicenter study. Ann Emerg Med 1993;22:579–82.

[9] Goldman L, Kirtane AJ. Triage of patients with acute chest pain and possible cardiac ischemia: the elusive search for diagnostic perfection. Ann Intern Med 2003;139:987–95.

[10] Pope JH, Aufderheide TP, Ruthazer R, et al. Missed diagnosis of acute cardiac ischemia in the emergency department. N Engl J Med 2000;342:1163–70.

[11] Canto JG, Shlipak MG, Roger WJ, et al. Prevalence, clinical characteristics, and mortality among patients with myocardial infarction presenting without chest pain. JAMA 2000;283: 3223–9.

[12] Rude RE, Poole WK, Muller J, et al. Electrocardiographic and clinical criteria for recognition of acute myocardial infarction based on analysis of 3,697 patients. Am J Cardiol 1983;52:936–42.

[13] Fesmire FM, Percy RF, Wears RL, et al. Initial ECG in Q wave and non-Q wave myocardial infarction. Ann Emerg Med 1989;18:741–6.

[14] Rouan GW, Lee TH, Cook EF, et al. Clinical characteristics and outcome of acute myocardial infarction in patients with initially normal or nonspecific electrocardiograms (a report from the Multicenter Chest Pain Study). Am J Cardiol 1989;64:1087–92.

[15] Brady WJ. ST segment elevation in ED adult chest pain patients: etiology and diagnostic accuracy for AMI. J Emerg Med 1998;16:797–8.

[16] Otto LA, Aufderheide TP. Evaluation of ST segment elevation criteria for the prehospital electrocardiographic diagnosis of acute myocardial infarction. Ann Emerg Med 1994;23: 17–24.

[17] Surawicz B, Parikh SR. Prevalence of male and female patterns of early ventricular repolarization in the normal ECG of males and females from childhood to old age. J Am Coll Cardiol 2002;40:1870–6.

[18] Wang K, Asinger RW, Marriott HJ. ST segment elevation in conditions other than acute myocardial infarction. N Engl J Med 2003;349:2128–35.

[19] Karlson BW, Herlitz J, Wiklund O, et al. Early prediction of acute myocardial infarction from clinical history, examination and electrocardiogram in the emergency room. Am J Cardiol 1991;68:171–5.

[20] Braunwald E, Jones RH, Mark DB, et al. Diagnosing and managing unstable angina. Agency for Health Care Policy and Research. Circulation 1994;90:613–22.

[21] Brush JE, Brand DA, Acampora D, et al. Use of the initial electrocardiogram to predict in-hospital complications of acute myocardial infarction. N Engl J Med 1985;312: 1137–41.

[22] Zalenski RJ, Sloan EP, Chen EH, et al. The emergency department ECG and immediately life-threatening complications in initially uncomplicated suspected myocardial ischemia. Ann Emerg Med 1988;17:221–6.

[23] Zalenski RJ, Rydman RJ, Sloan EP, et al. The emergency department electrocardiogram and hospital complications in myocardial infarction patients. Acad Emerg Med 1996;3: 318–25.

[24] McCarthy BD, Wong JB, Selker HP. Detecting acute cardiac ischemia in the emergency department: a review of the literature. J Gen Intern Med 1990;5:365–73.

[25] Karlson BW, Herlitz J. Hospitalisations, infarct development, and mortality in patients with chest pain and a normal admission electrocardiogram in relation to gender. Coron Artery Dis 1996;7:231–7.

[26] Welch RD, Zalenski RJ, Frederick PD, et al. Prognostic value of a normal or nonspecific initial electrocardiogram in acute myocardial infarction. JAMA 2001;286:1977–84.

[27] Fesmire FM, Percy RF, Bardoner JB, et al. Usefulness of automated serial 12-lead ECG monitoring during the initial emergency department evaluation of patients with chest pain. Ann Emerg Med 1998;31:3–11.

[28] Kudenchuk PJ, Maynard C, Cobb LA, et al. Utility of the prehospital electrocardiogram in diagnosing acute coronary syndromes. J Am Coll Cardiol 1998;32:17–27.

[29] Raitt MH, Maynard C, Wagner GS, et al. Appearance of abnormal Q waves early in the course of acute myocardial infarction: implications for efficacy of thrombolytic therapy. J Am Coll Cardiol 1995;25:1084–8.

[30] Bar FW, Volders PG, Hoppener B, et al. Development of ST segment elevation and Q- and R-wave changes in acute myocardial infarction and the influence of thrombolytic therapy. Am J Cardiol 1996;77:337–43.

[31] Mills RM, Young E, Gorlin R, et al. Natural history of S-T segment elevation after acute myocardial infarction. Am J Cardiol 1975;35:609–14.

[32] Chou TC, Knilans TK. Electrocardiography in clinical practice. Philadelphia: WB Saunders Co.; 1996.

[33] Soo CS. Tall precordial T waves with depressed ST take-off: an early sign of acute myocardial infarction? Singapore Med J 1995;36:236–7.

[34] Smith SW, Zvosec DL, Henry TD, et al. The ECG in acute MI: an evidence-based manual of reperfusion therapy. Philadelphia: Lippincott, Williams, and Wilkins; 2002. p. 358.

[35] Dressler W, Roesler H. High T waves in the earliest stage of myocardial infarction. Am Heart J 1947;34:627–45.

[36] Freundlich J. The diagnostic significance of tall upright T waves in the chest leads. Am Heart J 1956;52:749–67.

[37] Pinto IJ, Nanda NC, Biswas AK, et al. Tall upright T waves in the precordial leads. Circulation 1967;36:708–16.

[38] Smith FM. The ligation of coronary arteries with electrocardiographic study. Arch Intern Med 1918;5:1–27.

[39] Bohning A, Katz LN. Unusual changes in the electrocardiograms of patients with recent coronary occlusion. Am J Med Sci 1933;186:39–52.

[40] Wood FC, Wolferth CC. Huge T waves in precordial leads in cardiac infarction. Am Heart J 1934;9:706–21.
[41] Bayley RH, LaDue JS, York DJ. Electrocardiographic changes (local ventricular ischemia and injury) produced in the dog by temporary occlusion of a coronary artery, showing a new stage in the evolution of myocardial infarction. Am Heart J 1944;27:164–9.
[42] Graham GK, Laforet EG. An electrocardiographic and morphologic study of changes following ligation of the left coronary artery in human beings: a report of two cases. Am Heart J 1952;43:42–52.
[43] Wachtel FW, Teich EM. Tall precordial T waves as the earliest sign in diaphragmatic wall infarction. Am Heart J 1956;51:917–20.
[44] Blomkalns AL, Gibler WB, Chenier TC, et al. Identification of ECG abnormalities associated with positive cardiac markers in the evaluation of patients with acute chest pain. Acad Emerg Med 2001;8:551–2.
[45] Hochrein J, Sun F, Pieper KS, et al. Higher T wave amplitude associated with better prognosis in patients receiving thrombolytic therapy for acute myocardial infarction (a GUSTO-1 substudy). Global utilization of streptokinase and tissue plasminogen activator for occluded coronary arteries. Am J Cardiol 1998;81:1078–84.
[46] Wilkins ML, Pryor AD, Maynard C, et al. An electrocardiographic acuteness score for quantifying the timing of a myocardial infarction to guide decisions regarding reperfusion therapy. Am J Cardiol 1995;75:617–20.
[47] Corey KE, Maynard C, Pahlm O, et al. Combined historical and electrocardiographic timing of acute anterior and inferior myocardial infarcts for prediction of reperfusion achievable size limitation. Am J Cardiol 1999;83:826–31.
[48] Herz I, Birnbaum Y, Zlotikamien B, et al. The prognostic implications of negative T waves in the leads with ST segment elevation on admission in acute myocardial infarction. Cardiology 1999;92:121–7.
[49] Smith SW. ST elevation in anterior acute myocardial infarction differs with different methods of measurement [abstract]. Acad Emerg Med 2003;10:560.
[50] Willems JL, Willems RJ, Willems GM, et al. Significance of initial ST segment elevation and depression for the management of thrombolytic therapy in acute myocardial infarction. Circulation 1990;82:1147–58.
[51] Bush HS, Ferguson JJ, Angelini P, et al. Twelve-lead electrocardiographic evaluation of ischemia during percutaneous transluminal coronary angioplasty and its correlation with acute reocclusion. Am Heart J 1991;121:1591–9.
[52] Tamura A, Mikuriya Y, Kataoka H, et al. Emergent coronary angiographic findings of patients with ST depression in the inferior or lateral leads, or both, during anterior wall acute myocardial infarction. Am J Cardiol 1995;76(A):516–7.
[53] Bell JB, Leibrandt PN, Greenfield JC, et al. Comparison of an automated thrombolytic predictive instrument to both diagnostic software and an expert cardiologist for diagnosis of an ST elevation acute myocardial infarction. J Electrocardiol 2000;33(Suppl):259–62.
[54] Massel D, Dawdy JA, Melendez LJ. Strict reliance on a computer algorithm or measurable ST segment criteria may lead to errors in thrombolytic therapy eligibility. Am Heart J 2000;140:221–6.
[55] Prineas J, Crow RS, Blackburn H. The Minnesota Code Manual of Electrocardiographic Findings: Standards and procedures for measurement and classification. Littleton, MA: John Wright, PSG, Inc.; 1982.
[56] GISSI (Gruppo Italiano Per Lo Studio Della Sopravivenza Nell'Infarto Miocardio). Effectiveness of intravenous thrombolytic treatment in acute myocardial infarction. Lancet 1986;1:397–401.
[57] Chesebro JH, Knatterud G, Roberts R, et al. Thrombolysis in Myocardial Infarction (TIMI) Trial, Phase I: a comparison between intravenous tissue plasminogen activator and intravenous streptokinase: clinical findings through hospital discharge. Circulation 1987;76:142–54.

[58] ISIS-2 (Second International Study of Infarct Survival) Collaborative Group. Randomised trial of intravenous streptokinase, oral aspirin, both, or neither among 17,187 cases of suspected acute myocardial infarction: ISIS-2. Lancet 1988;2:349–60.

[59] GISSI-2 (Gruppo Italiano Per Lo Studio Della Sopravivenza Nell'Infarto Miocardio). GISSI-2: a factorial randomised trial of alteplase versus streptokinase and heparin versus no heparin among 12,490 patients with acute myocardial infarction. Lancet 1990;336: 65–71.

[60] ISIS-3 (Third International Study of Infarct Survival) Collaborative Study Group. ISIS-3: a randomised comparison of streptokinase versus tissue plasminogen activator vs anistreplase and of aspirin plus heparin vs aspirin alone among 41,299 cases of suspected acute myocardial infarction. Lancet 1992;339:753–70.

[61] TIMI III A. Early effects of tissue-type plasminogen activator added to conventional therapy on the culprit coronary lesion in patients presenting with ischemic cardiac pain at rest. Results of the Thrombolysis in Myocardial Ischemia TIMI (Thrombolysis in Myocardial Infarction) IIIA trial. Circulation 1993;87:38–52.

[62] Ryan TJ, Antman EM, Brooks NH, et al. 1999 update: ACC/AHA guidelines for the management of patients with acute myocardial infarction. J Am Coll Cardiol 1999;34:890–911.

[63] Joint European Society of Cardiology/American College of Cardiology Committee. Myocardial infarction redefined: a consensus document of the Joint European Society of Cardiology/American College of Cardiology committee for the redefinition of myocardial infarction. J Am Coll Cardiol 2000;36:959–69.

[64] Smith SW. Upwardly concave ST segment morphology is common in acute left anterior descending coronary artery occlusion [abstract]. Acad Emerg Med 2003;10:516.

[65] Kosuge M, Kimura K, Ishikawa T, et al. Value of ST segment elevation pattern in predicting infarct size and left ventricular function at discharge in patients with reperfused acute anterior myocardial infarction. Am Heart J 1999;137:522–7.

[66] Clements IP. The electrocardiogram in acute myocardial infarction. Armonk, NY: Futura Publishing Co., Inc.; 1998.

[67] Adams J, Trent R, Rawles JM, on behalf of the GREAT Group. Earliest electrocardiographic evidence of myocardial infarction: implication for thrombolytic treatment. BMJ 1993;307:409–13.

[68] Menown IB, Mackenzie G, Adgey AA. Optimizing the initial 12-lead electrocardiographic diagnosis of acute myocardial infarction. Eur Heart J 2000;21:275–83.

[69] Kudenchuk PJ, Ho MT, Weaver WD, et al. Accuracy of computer-interpreted electrocardiography in selecting patients for thrombolytic therapy. J Am Coll Card 1991;17:1486–91.

[70] Selker HP, Beshansky JR, Griffith JL. Use of the electrocardiograph-based thrombolytic predictive instrument to assist thrombolytic and reperfusion therapy for acute myocardial infarction. A multicenter, randomized, controlled, clinical effectiveness trial. Ann Intern Med 2002;137:87–95.

[71] Sharkey SW, Berger CR, Brunette DD, et al. Impact of the electrocardiogram on the delivery of thrombolytic therapy for acute myocardial infarction. Am J Cardiol 1994;73:550–3.

[72] Smith SW. T wave amplitude to QRS amplitude ratio best distinguishes the ST elevation of anterior left ventricular aneurysm from anterior acute myocardial infarction. Acad Emerg Med 2003;10:516–7.

[73] Smith SW, Khalil A, Heller K, et al. R wave amplitude distinguishes early repolarization from subtle anterior STEMI. Acad Emerg Med 2005;12(Suppl 5):132.

[74] Huey BL, Beller GA, Kaiser D, et al. A comprehensive analysis of myocardial infarction due to left circumflex artery occlusion: comparison with infarction due to right coronary artery and left anterior descending artery occlusion. J Am Coll Cardiol 1988;12: 1156–66.

[75] Berry C, Zalewsky A, Kovach R, et al. Surface electrocardiogram in the detection of transmural myocardial ischemia during coronary artery occlusion. Am J Cardiol 1989; 63:21–6.

[76] Veldkamp RF, Sawchak S, Pope JE, et al. Performance of an automated real-time ST segment analysis program to detect coronary occlusion and reperfusion. J Electrocardiol 1996; 29:257–63.

[77] Christian TF, Clements IP, Gibbons RJ. Noninvasive identification of myocardium at risk in patients with acute myocardial infarction and nondiagnostic electrocardiograms with technetium-99m-sestamibi. Circulation 1991;83:1615–20.

[78] O'Keefe JHJ, Sayed-Taha K, Gibson W, et al. Do patients with left circumflex coronary artery-related acute myocardial infarction without ST segment elevation benefit from reperfusion therapy? [comments]. Am J Cardiol 1995;75:718–20.

[79] Christian TF, Gibbons RJ, Clements IP, et al. Estimates of myocardium at risk and collateral flow in acute myocardial infarction using electrocardiographic indexes with comparison to radionuclide and angiographic measures. J Am Coll Cardiol 1995;26:388–93.

[80] Hands ME, Lloyd BL, Robinson JS, et al. Prognostic significance of electrocardiographic site of infarction after correction for enzymatic size of infarction. Circulation 1986;73: 885–91.

[81] Stone PH, Raabe DS, Jaffe AS, et al. Prognostic significance of location and type of MI: independent adverse outcome associated with anterior location. J Am Coll Cardiol 1988; 11:453–63.

[82] Mauri F, Gasparini M, Barbonaglia L, et al. Prognostic significance of the extent of myocardial injury in acute myocardial infarction treated by streptokinase (the GISSI Trial). Am J Cardiol 1989;63:1291–5.

[83] Bar FW, Vermeer F, de Zwaan C, et al. Value of admission electrocardiogram in predicting outcome of thrombolytic therapy in acute myocardial infarction. Am J Cardiol 1987;59: 6–13.

[84] Lee KL, Woodlief LH, Topol EJ, et al. Predictors of 30-day mortality in the era of reperfusion for acute myocardial infarction: results from an international trial of 41,021 patients. Circulation 1995;91:1659–68.

[85] Savonitto S, Ardissino D, Granger CB, et al. Prognostic value of the admission electrocardiogram in acute coronary syndromes. JAMA 1999;281:707–13.

[86] Birnbaum Y, Herz I, Sclarovsky S, et al. Prognostic significance of the admission electrocardiogram in acute myocardial infarction. J Am Coll Cardiol 1996;27:1128–32.

[87] Hyde TA, French JK, Wong CK, et al. Four-year survival of patients with acute coronary syndromes without ST segment elevation and prognostic significance of 0.5-mm ST segment depression. Am J Cardiol 1999;84:379–85.

[88] Kaul P, Newby LK, Fu Y, et al. Troponin T and quantitative ST segment depression offer complementary prognostic information in the risk stratification of acute coronary syndrome patients. J Am Coll Cardiol 2003;41:371–80.

[89] Ellestad MH, Crump R, Surbur M. The significance of lead strength on ST changes during treadmill stress tests. J Electrocardiol 1992;25(Suppl):31–4.

[90] Hollenberg M, Go JJ, Massie BM, et al. Influence of R wave amplitude on exercise-induced ST depression: need for a "gain factor" correlation when interpreting stress electrocardiograms. Am J Cardiol 1985;56:13.

[91] Hakki AH, Iskandrian SD, Kutalek, et al. R wave amplitude: a new determinant of failure of patients with coronary heart disease to manifest ST segment depression during exercise. J Am Coll Cardiol 1984;3:1155.

[92] Santinga JT, Brymer JF, Smith F, et al. The influence of lead strength on the ST changes with exercise electrocardiography (correlative study with coronary arteriography). J Electrocardiol 1977;10:387.

[93] Lee HS, Cross SJ, Rawles JM, et al. Patients with suspected myocardial infarction who present with ST depression. Lancet 1993;342:1204–7.

[94] Wong PS, el Gaylani N, Griffith K, et al. The clinical course of patients with acute myocardial infarction who are unsuitable for thrombolytic therapy because of the presenting electrocardiogram. UK Heart Attack Study Investigators. Coron Artery Dis 1998;9:747–52.

[95] Diderholm E, Andren B, Frostfeldt G, et al. ST depression in ECG at entry indicates severe coronary lesions and large benefits of an early invasive treatment strategy in unstable coronary artery disease; the FRISC II ECG substudy. The Fast Revascularisation during In-Stability in Coronary artery disease. Eur Heart J 2002;23:41–9.

[96] Fibrinolytic Therapy Trialists' (FTT) Collaborative Group. Indications for fibrinolytic therapy in suspected acute myocardial infarction: collaborative overview of early mortality and major morbidity results from all randomised trials of more than 1000 patients. Lancet 1994;343:311–22.

[97] Anderson HV, Cannon CP, Stone PH, et al. One-year results of the Thrombolysis in Myocardial Infarction (TIMI) IIIB clinical trial. A randomised comparison of tissue-type plasminogen activator versus placebo and early invasive versus early conservative strategies in unstable angina and non-Q wave myocardial infarction. J Am Coll Cardiol 1995;26: 1643–50.

[98] Ryan TJ, Anderson JL, Antman EM, et al. ACC/AHA guidelines for the management of patients with acute myocardial infarction: a report of the American College of Cardiology/American Heart Association Task Force on Practice Guidelines (Committee on Management of Acute Myocardial Infarction). J Am Coll Cardiol 1996;28: 1328–428.

[99] Cragg DR, Friedman HZ, Bonema JD, et al. Outcome of patients with acute myocardial infarction who are ineligible for thrombolytic therapy. Ann Intern Med 1991;115: 173–7.

[100] Rowlandson I, Kudenchuk PJ, Elko P. Computerized recognition of acute infarction. Criteria advances and test results. J Electrocardiol 1990;23(Suppl):1–5.

[101] Elko P, Weaver WD, Kudenchuk PJ, Rowlandson I. The dilemma of sensitivity versus specificity in computer-interpreted acute myocardial infarction. J Electrocardiol 1992; 24(Suppl):2–7.

[102] Elko P, Rowlandson I. A statistical analysis of the ECG measurements used in computerized interpretation of acute anterior myocardial infarction with applications to interpretive criteria development. J Electrocardiol 1993;25(Suppl):113–9.

[103] Tighe M, Kellett J, Corry E, et al. The early diagnosis of acute myocardial infarction. Comparison of a simple algorithm with a computer program for electrocardiogram interpretation. Irish J Med Sci 1996;165:159–63.

[104] Brady WJ, Perron AD, Syverud SA, et al. Reciprocal ST segment depression: impact on the electrocardiographic diagnosis of ST segment elevation acute myocardial infarction. Am J Emerg Med 2002;20:35–8.

[105] Birnbaum Y, Sclarovsky S, Solodky A, et al. Prediction of the level of left anterior descending coronary artery obstruction during anterior wall acute myocardial infarction by the admission electrocardiogram. Am J Cardiol 1993;72:823–6.

[106] Tamura A, Kataoka H, Mikuriya Y, et al. Inferior ST segment depression as a useful marker for identifying proximal left anterior descending artery occlusion during acute anterior myocardial infarction. Eur Heart J 1995b;16:1795–9.

[107] Engelen DJ, Gorgens AP, Cheriex EC, et al. Value of the electrocardiogram in localizing the occlusion site in the left anterior descending coronary artery in acute myocardial infarction. J Am Coll Cardiol 1999;34:389–95.

[108] Kosuge M, Kimura K, Toshiyuki I, et al. Electrocardiographic criteria for predicting total occlusion of the proximal left anterior descending coronary artery in anterior wall acute myocardial infarction. Clin Cardiol 2001;24:33–8.

[109] Peterson ED, Hathaway WR, Zabel KM, et al. Prognostic significance of precordial ST segment depression during inferior myocardial infarction in the thrombolytic era: results in 16,521 patients. J Am Coll Cardiol 1996;28:305–12.

[110] Goldberger AL, Erickson R. Subtle ECG sign of acute infarction: prominent reciprocal ST depression with minimal primary ST elevation. Pacing Clin Electrophysiol 1981; 4:709–12.

[111] de Zwaan C, Bar FW, Janssen JHA, et al. Angiographic and clinical characteristics of patients with unstable angina showing an ECG pattern indicating critical narrowing of the proximal LAD coronary artery. Am Heart J 1989;117:657–65.

[112] de Zwaan C, Bar FW, Wellens HJJ. Characteristic electrocardiographic pattern indicating a critical stenosis high in left anterior descending coronary artery in patients admitted because of impending myocardial infarction. Am Heart J 1982;103:730–6.

[113] Oliva PB, Hammill SC, Edwards WD. Electrocardiographic diagnosis of postinfarction regional pericarditis: ancillary observations regarding the effect of reperfusion on the rapidity and amplitude of T-wave inversion after acute myocardial infarction. Circulation 1993;88: 896–904.

[114] Doevendans PA, Gorgels AP, van der Zee R, et al. Electrocardiographic diagnosis of reperfusion during thrombolytic therapy in acute myocardial infarction. Am J Cardiol 1995;75: 1206–10.

[115] Wehrens XH, Doevendans PA, Ophuis TJ, et al. A comparison of electrocardiographic changes during reperfusion of acute myocardial infarction by thrombolysis or percutaneous transluminal coronary angioplasty. Am Heart J 2000;139:430–6.

[116] Goldberger AL. Myocardial infarction: electrocardiographic differential diagnosis. St. Louis: Mosby; 1991. p. 386.

[117] Friedman HH, editor. Diagnostic electrocardiography and vectorcardiography. New York: McGraw-Hill; 1985.

[118] Haines DE, Raabe DS, Gundel WD, et al. Anatomic and prognostic significance of new T-wave inversion in unstable angina. Am J Cardiol 1983;52:14–8.

[119] Tandy TK, Bottomy DP, Lewis J. Wellens' syndrome. Ann Emerg Med 1999;33: 347–51.

[120] Prinzmetal M, Shaw CM, Maxwell MH. Studies on the mechanism of ventricular activity. VI. The depolarization complex in pure subendocardial infarction: role of the sub-endocardial region in the normal electrocardiogram. Am J Med 1954;16:469–88.

[121] Moon JCC, De Arenaza DP, Elkington AG, et al. The pathologic basis of Q wave and non-Q wave myocardial infarction. J Am Coll Cardiol 2004;44:554–60.

[122] Phibbs B. "Transmural" versus "subendocardial" myocardial infarction: an electrocardiographic myth. J Am Coll Cardiol 1983;1:561–4.

[123] Fuster V, Badimon L, Badimon JJ, et al. The pathogenesis of coronary artery disease and the acute coronary syndromes (1). N Engl J Med 1992;326:242–50.

[124] Theroux P, Fuster V. Acute coronary syndromes: unstable angina and non-Q wave myocardial infarction. Circulation 1998;97:1195–206.

[125] Phibbs B, Marcus F, Marriott HJ, et al. Q wave versus non-Q wave myocardial infarction: a meaningless distinction. J Am Coll Cardiol 1999;33:576–82.

[126] Krone RJ, Greenberg H, Dwyer EMJ, et al. Long-term prognostic significance of ST segment depression during acute myocardial infarction. The Multicenter Diltiazem Postinfarction Trial Research Group. J Am Coll Cardiol 1993;22:361–7.

[127] Barold SS, Falkoff MD, Ong LS, et al. Significance of transient electrocardiographic Q waves in coronary artery disease. Cardiol Clin 1987;5:367–80.

[128] Kleiger RE, Boden WE, Schechtman KB, et al. Frequency and significance of late evolution of Q waves in patients with initial non-Q wave acute myocardial infarction. Diltiazem Reinfarction Study Group. Am J Cardiol 1990;65:23–7.

[129] Kaplan BM, Berkson DM. Serial electrocardiograms after myocardial infarction. Ann Intern Med 1964;60:430–5.

[130] Blanke H, Scherff F, Karsch KR, et al. Electrocardiographic changes after streptokinase-induced recanalization in patients with acute left anterior descending artery obstruction. Circulation 1983;68:406–12.

[131] Claeys MJ, Bosmans J, Veenstra L, et al. Determinants and prognostic implications of persistent ST segment elevation after primary angioplasty for acute myocardial infarction:

importance of microvascular reperfusion injury on clinical outcome. Circulation 1999;99: 1972–7.

[132] Krucoff MW, Croll MA, Pope JE, et al. Continuous 12-lead ST segment recovery analysis in the TAMI 7 study. Performance of a non-invasive method for real-time detection of failed myocardial reperfusion. Circulation 1993;88:437–46.

[133] Kusniec J, Slolodky A, Strasberg B, et al. The relationship between the electrocardiographic pattern with TIMI flow class and ejection fraction in patients with first acute anterior wall myocardial infarction. Eur Heart J 1997;18:420–5.

[134] Levin DC, Harrington DP, Bettmann MA, et al. Anatomic variation of the coronary arteries supplying the anterolateral aspect of the left ventricle: possible explanation of the unexplained anterior aneurysm. Invest Radiol 1982;17:458–62.

[135] Tamura A, Kataoka H, Nagase K, et al. Clinical significance of inferior ST elevation during acute anterior myocardial infarction. Br Heart J 1995;74:611–4.

[136] Porter A, Wyshelesky A, Strasberg B, et al. Correlation between the admission electrocardiogram and regional wall motion abnormalities as detected by echocardiography in anterior acute myocardial infarction. Cardiology 2000;94:118–26.

[137] Assali AR, Sclarovsky S, Herz I, et al. Comparison of patients with inferior wall acute myocardial infarction with versus without ST segment elevation in leads V5 and V6. Am J Cardiol 1998;81:81–3.

[138] Agarwal JB, Khaw K, Aurignac F, et al. Importance of posterior chest leads in patients with suspected myocardial infarction, but nondiagnostic, routine 12-lead electrogram. Am J Cardiol 1999;83:323–6.

[139] Shah A, Wagner GS, Califf RM, et al. Comparative prognostic significance of simultaneous versus independent resolution of ST segment depression relative to ST segment elevation during acute myocardial infarction. J Am Coll Cardiol 1997;30:1478–83.

[140] Kulkarni AU, Brown R, Ayoubi M, et al. Clinical use of posterior electrocardiographic leads: a prospective electrocardiographic analysis during coronary occlusion. Am Heart J 1996;131:736–41.

[141] Roul G, Bareiss P, Germain P, et al. Isolated ST segment depression from V2 to V4 leads, an early electrocardiographic sign of posterior myocardial infarction. Arch Mal Coeur Vaiss 1991;84:1815–9.

[142] Oraii S, Maleki I, Tavakolian AA, et al. Prevalence and outcome of ST segment elevation in posterior electrocardiographic leads during acute myocardial infarction. J Electrocardiol 1999;32:275–8.

[143] Melendez LJ, Jones DT, Salcedo JR. Usefulness of three additional electrocardiographic chest leads (V7, V8, V9) in the diagnosis of acute myocardial infarction. Can Med Assoc J 1978;119:745–8.

[144] Wung SF, Drew BJ. New electrocardiographic criteria for posterior wall acute myocardial ischemia validated by a percutaneous transluminal coronary angioplasty model of acute myocardial infarction. Am J Cardiol 2001;87(A4):970–4.

[145] Matetzky S, Freimark D, Chouraqui P, et al. Significance of ST segment elevations in posterior chest leads (V7–V9) in patients with acute inferior myocardial infarction: application for thrombolytic therapy. J Am Coll Cardiol 1998;31:506–11.

[146] Zalenski RJ, Rydman RJ, Sloan EP, et al. Value of posterior and right ventricular leads in comparison to the standard 12-lead electrocardiogram in evaluation of ST segment elevation in suspected acute myocardial infarction. Am J Cardiol 1997;79:1579–85.

[147] Brady WJ, Hwang V, Sullivan R. A comparison of 12- and 15-lead ECGs in ED chest pain patients: impact on diagnosis, therapy, and disposition. Am J Emerg Med 2000; 18:239–43.

[148] Zimetbaum PJ, Krishnan S, Gold A, et al. Usefulness of ST segment elevation in lead III exceeding that of lead II for identifying the location of the totally occluded coronary artery in inferior wall myocardial infarction. Am J Cardiol 1998;81:918–9.

[149] Chia BL, Yip JW, Tan HC, et al. Usefulness of ST elevation II/III ratio and ST deviation in lead I for identifying the culprit artery in inferior wall acute myocardial infarction. Am J Cardiol 2000;86:341–3.

[150] Bairey CN, Shah PK, Lew AS, et al. Electrocardiographic differentiation of occlusion of the left circumflex versus the right coronary artery as a cause of inferior acute myocardial infarction. Am J Cardiol 1987;60:456–9.

[151] Herz I, Assali AR, Adler Y, et al. New electrocardiographic criteria for predicting either the right or left circumflex artery as the culprit coronary artery in inferior wall acute myocardial infarction. Am J Cardiol 1997;80:1343–5.

[152] Geft IL, Shah PK, Rodriguez L, et al. ST elevations in leads V1 to V5 may be caused by right coronary artery occlusion and acute right ventricular infarction. Am J Cardiol 1984;53: 991–6.

[153] Hasdai D, Sclarovsky S, Solodky A, et al. Prognostic significance of maximal precordial ST segment depression in right (V1 to V3) versus left (V4 to V6) leads in patients with inferior wall acute myocardial infarction. Am J Cardiol 1994;74:1081–4.

[154] Shah PK, Pichler M, Berman DS, et al. Noninvasive identification of a high risk subset of patients with acute myocardial infarction. Am J Cardiol 1980;46:915–21.

[155] Zehender M, Kasper W, Schonthaler M, et al. Right ventricular infarction as an independent predictor of prognosis after acute inferior myocardial infarction. N Engl J Med 1993; 328:981–8.

[156] Zehender M, Kasper W, Kauder E, et al. Eligibility for and benefit of thrombolytic therapy in inferior myocardial infarction: focus on the prognostic importance of right ventricular infarction. J Am Coll Cardiol 1994;24:362–9.

[157] Bowers TR, O'Neill WW, Grines CL, et al. Effect of reperfusion on biventricular function and survival after right ventricular infarction. N Engl J Med 1998;338:933–40.

[158] Andersen HR, Neilson D, Lund O, et al. Prognostic significance of right ventricular infarction; diagnosed by ST elevation in right chest leads V3R to V7R. Int J Cardiol 1989;23: 349–56.

[159] Kopelman HA, Forman MB, Wilson H, et al. Right ventricular myocardial infarction in patients with chronic lung disease: possible role of right ventricular hypertrophy. J Am Coll Cardiol 1985;5:1302–7.

[160] Lopez-Sendon J, Coma-Canella I, Alcasena S, et al. Electrocardiographic findings in acute right ventricular infarction: sensitivity and specificity of electrocardiographic alterations in right precordial leads V4R, V3R, V1, V2, and V3. J Am Coll Cardiol 1985;6:1273–9.

[161] Andersen HR, Nielsen D, Hanse LG. The normal right chest electrocardiogram. J Electrocardiol 1987;20:27–32.

[162] Simon R, Angehrn W. Right ventricular involvement in infero-posterior myocardial infarct: clinical significance of ECG diagnosis. Schweiz Med Wochenschr 1993;123:1499–507.

[163] Go AS, Barron HV, Rundle AC, et al. Bundle-branch block and in-hospital mortality in acute myocardial infarction. National Registry of Myocardial Infarction. Ann Intern Med 1998;129:690–7.

[164] Newby KH, Pisano O, Krucoff MW, et al. Incidence and clinical relevance of the occurrence of bundle-branch block in patients treated with thrombolytic therapy. Circulation 1996;94:2424–8.

[165] Waxman DA, Smith SW, Kontos MC, et al. Beyond left bundle-branch block: looking for the acute transmural myocardial infarction. Ann Emerg Med 2002;39:94–8.

[166] Sgarbossa EB, Pinski SL, Barbagelata A, et al. Electrocardiographic diagnosis of evolving acute myocardial infarction in the presence of left bundle-branch block. N Engl J Med 1996; 334:481–7.

[167] Sgarbossa EB, Pinski SL, Topol EJ, et al. Acute myocardial infarction and complete bundle branch block at hospital admission: clinical characteristics and outcome in the thrombolytic era. J Am Coll Cardiol 1998;31:105–10.

[168] Edhouse JA, Sakr M, Angus J, et al. Suspected myocardial infarction and left bundle branch block: electrocardiographic indicators of acute ischaemia. J Accident Emerg Med 1999;16:331–5.

[169] Kontos MC, McQueen RH, Jesse RL, et al. Can myocardial infarction be rapidly identified in emergency department patients who have left bundle branch block? Ann Emerg Med 2001;37:431–8.

[170] Wackers FJT. The diagnosis of myocardial infarction in the presence of left bundle branch block. Cardiol Clin 1987;5:393–401.

[171] Stark KS, Krucoff MW, Schryver B, et al. Quantification of ST segment changes during coronary angioplasty in patients with left bundle branch block. Am J Cardiol 1991;67: 1219–22.

[172] Fesmire FM. ECG diagnosis of acute myocardial infarction in the presence of left bundle-branch block in patients undergoing continuous ECG monitoring. Ann Emerg Med 1995; 26:69–82.

ELSEVIER
SAUNDERS

EMERGENCY
MEDICINE
CLINICS OF
NORTH AMERICA

Emerg Med Clin N Am 24 (2006) 91–111

ST Segment and T Wave Abnormalities Not Caused by Acute Coronary Syndromes

William J. Brady, MD

*Department of Emergency Medicine, University of Virginia School of Medicine,
Charlottesville, VA 22911, USA*

The evaluation of the chest pain patient suspected of acute coronary syndrome (ACS) represents the major indication for electrocardiograph (ECG) performance in the emergency department (ED) and prehospital settings [1]. The ECG demonstrates significant abnormality in a minority of these patients, ranging from minimal nonspecific ST segment/T wave changes to pronounced STE and T wave abnormalities, including the prominent T wave, the inverted T wave, and the nonspecific T wave (Figs. 1 and 2). The ECG syndromes responsible for these various abnormalities include potentially malignant entities, such as ACS and cardiomyopathy, and less concerning patterns, such as benign early repolarization (BER) or ventricular paced rhythms (VPR) [2–4].

In a study considering all chest pain patients with electrocardiographic ST segment depression (STD), the following clinical syndromes were responsible for the ECG abnormality: ACS, 26%; left ventricular hypertrophy (LVH), 43%; bundle branch block (BBB), 21%; VPR, 5%; left ventricular aneurysm, 3%; and other patterns, 1% [5]. Similarly, STE is a fairly common finding on the ECG of the chest pain patient and frequently does not indicate STE acute myocardial infarction (AMI). One prehospital study of adult chest pain patients revealed that, of patients manifesting STE who met criteria for fibrinolysis, most were not diagnosed with AMI; rather, LVH and left BBB were found more frequently [6]. Furthermore, in two reviews of adult ED chest pain patients with STE on ECG, the ST segment abnormality resulted from AMI in only 15%–31% of these populations; LVH, seen in 28%–30% of these patients, was a frequent cause of this STE. Other findings responsible for this STE included BER, acute

---

E-mail address: wb4z@virgnia.edu

doi:10.1016/j.emc.2005.08.004   *emed.theclinics.com*

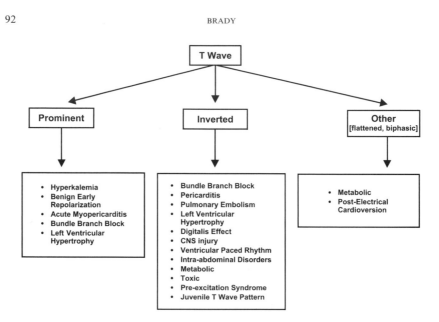

Fig. 1. Electrocardiographic differential diagnosis of T wave abnormalities—prominent, inverted, and nonspecific in non-ACS syndromes.

myopericarditis, BBB, VPR, and ventricular aneurysm [7,8]. In a critical care unit setting, Miller et al [9] showed that STE was noted frequently, yet was responsible for AMI in only 50% of patients.

This article discusses the non-ACS causes of ST segment/T wave abnormalities, highlighting differentiation from STE associated with ACS.

Benign early repolarization

BER is a normal electrocardiographic variant with no known association with cardiac dysfunction or disease. BER describes a pattern of STE with prominent T waves most often seen in the precordial leads. A recent investigation demonstrated a BER prevalence of 29% among patients undergoing a screening health examination. Patients who had early repolarization were more likely to be male, were younger (less than age 40 years), and tended to be more athletically active compared with those individuals without the early repolarization pattern. The long-term health of these patients who had BER was equivalent to the control population [10]. In another large study of BER, the mean age of patients was 39 years (range, 16–80 years); although the pattern was seen across this rather broad age range, it was encountered predominantly in patients less than age 50 years and rarely seen in individuals older than age 70 years [11]. The BER pattern is seen much more often in men than in women. BER is encountered most frequently in younger black men (20–40 years of age) [12].

The electrocardiographic characterization of the BER pattern (Figs. 3–5) includes the following features: STE [1]; concavity of the initial, upsloping

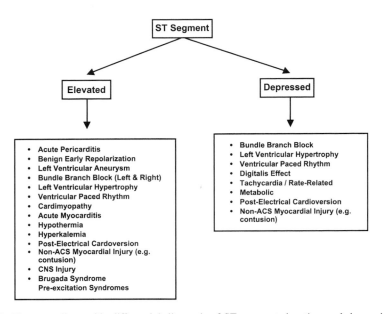

Fig. 2. Electrocardiographic differential diagnosis of ST segment elevation and depression in non-ACS syndromes.

portion of the ST segment [2]; notching or slurring of the J point [3]; symmetric, concordant, prominent T waves [4]; widespread distribution of the electrocardiographic abnormalities [5]; and temporal stability [6,13,14].

In the normal state, the ST segment is neither elevated nor depressed; it is located at the isoelectric baseline as defined by the TP segment. The ST segment itself begins at the J or juncture point. The ST segment is elevated in the BER pattern, usually less than 3.5 mm. The contour of the elevated ST segment is an important characteristic of the pattern; the ST segment seems to have been lifted off the baseline starting at the J point (Figs. 3–5). The normal concavity of the initial, upsloping portion of the ST segment is preserved. Eighty percent to 90% of individuals demonstrate STE less than 2 mm in the precordial leads and less than 0.5 mm in the limb leads; only 2% of cases of BER manifest STE greater than 5 mm [13,14]. In the BER pattern, the J point itself frequently is notched or irregular. This finding, although not diagnostic of BER, is highly suggestive of the diagnosis [11,13,15].

Prominent T waves also are encountered (see Figs. 3 and 4). These T wave are often of large amplitude and slightly asymmetric morphology. The T waves are concordant with the QRS complex (ie, oriented in the same direction as the major portion of the QRS complex) and usually are found in the precordial leads. The height of the T waves in BER ranges from approximately 6 mm in the precordial leads to 4–6 mm in the limb leads [11,13,16].

[1] ST segment elevation
[2] upward concavity of initial portion
     of ST segment
[3] notching or slurring of terminal
     QRS complex
[4] slightly asymmetric, concordant T
     waves of large amplitude
[5] widespread or diffuse distribution
     of ST segment elevation
[6] relative temporal stability

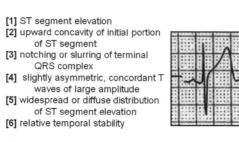

Fig. 3. ECG criteria for benign early repolarization.

These abnormalities are greatest in the precordial leads, particularly the precordial leads (leads V2–V5). STE in the limb leads, if present, is usually less pronounced. In fact, this isolated STE in the limb leads is seen in less than 10% of BER cases and should prompt consideration of another explanation for the observed ST segment abnormality, such as AMI. The T waves tend to follow the QRS complex in the BER pattern; essentially, pronounced STE usually is associated with prominent T waves in the same distribution.

Acute myopericarditis

Acute pericarditis is better termed acute myopericarditis in that both the pericardium and the superficial epicardium are inflamed. This epicardial inflammation produces the ST segment and related electrocardiographic changes; the pericardial membrane is electrically silent in a direct effect on the ST segment and T wave.

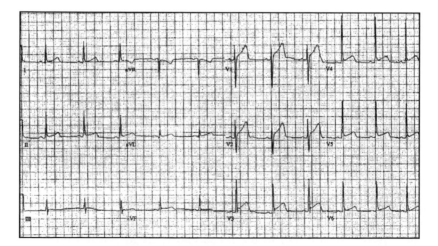

Fig. 4. Benign early repolarization.

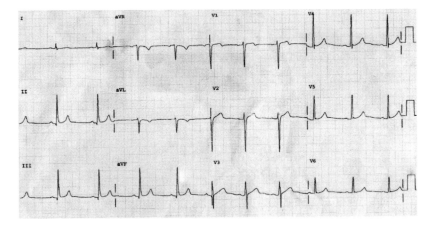

Fig. 5. Benign early repolarization.

The electrocardiographic abnormalities evolve through four classic stages (Fig. 6) [16]. Stage I (Figs. 6 and 7) is characterized by STE, prominent T waves, and (in most cases) PR segment depression. Stage II is characterized by a normalization of the initial abnormalities, namely a resolution of the STE. Stage III involves T wave inversion, usually in the same distribution where STE was encountered. Finally, stage IV is a normalization of all changes with a return to the baseline ECG. Persistent STE and pathologic Q waves are not encountered in patients who have myopericarditis—these electrocardiographic findings suggest another etiology.

These electrocardiographic stages usually occur in an unpredictable manner. In a general sense, stages I through III develop over hours to days. Conversely, changes related to stage IV myopericarditis may not develop for many days to many weeks. Furthermore, patients may not manifest all characteristic features. Finally, patients may present for medical care at a later stage of the process; for instance, the patient may present after a delay of

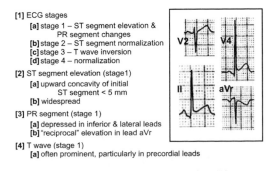

[1] ECG stages
  [a] stage 1 – ST segment elevation & PR segment changes
  [b] stage 2 – ST segment normalization
  [c] stage 3 – T wave inversion
  [d] stage 4 – normalization
[2] ST segment elevation (stage1)
  [a] upward concavity of initial ST segment < 5 mm
  [b] widespread
[3] PR segment (stage 1)
  [a] depressed in inferior & lateral leads
  [b] "reciprocal" elevation in lead aVr
[4] T wave (stage 1)
  [a] often prominent, particularly in precordial leads

Fig. 6. ECG criteria for myopericarditis.

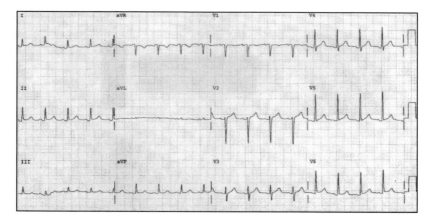

Fig. 7. Myopericarditis.

a week or more with chest discomfort and manifest electrocardiographic T wave inversion—the clinician having "missed" the STE.

Stage I abnormality—that is, STE, prominent T wave, and PR segment depression—is often electrocardiographically obvious with STE the most prominent electrocardiographic feature (Figs. 6 and 7). The magnitude of elevation usually ranges from 2–4 mm, with greater than 5 mm unusual for myopericarditis. The morphology of the elevated ST segment is most frequently concave in shape. In other cases, STE can also be obliquely flat or convex in contour; these morphologies, however, are suggestive of AMI [7]. STE resulting from myopericarditis is usually widespread, noted in the following electrocardiographic leads: I, II, III, aVL, aVF, and V2–V6—essentially all leads except the more rightward-oriented leads aVR and V1; reciprocal ST segment depression is seen in lead aVR and occasionally in lead V1. The STE is seen most often in many leads simultaneously, though it may be limited to a specific anatomic segment if the process is focal; if focal inflammation is present, the inferior wall most often is involved.

PR segment abnormality (Figs. 6 and 7) resulting from atrial inflammation and irritation is a highly suggestive feature of stage I myopericarditis. PR segment depression is described as "almost diagnostic" [16] and is best observed in the lateral precordial (V5 and V6) and inferior (II, III, and aVF) leads. Reciprocal PR segment elevation is seen in lead aVR; in many cases, this finding is in fact more obvious to the clinician compared with PR segment depression [17,18].

T wave inversion, a stage III feature, is usually transient and most often occurs in leads that had recently manifested stage I STE. The magnitude and morphology of the inverted T wave are nonspecific. The inverted T waves are usually of normal amplitude with symmetric initial (downsloping) and final (upsloping) limbs, which can be confused with an ACS presentation.

Additional electrocardiographic findings may be noted in the patient who presents with diseases associated with pericarditis: myocarditis and pericardial effusion. Myocarditis may manifest Q waves, bundle branch block, and dysrhythmias (Figs. 8 and 9). Electrocardiographic changes suggestive of pericardial effusion include widespread low voltage (resulting from increased resistance to injury current flow with the accumulated fluid) and electrical alternans (a beat-to-beat alteration in QRS complex size caused by shifting of the heart within the fluid-filled pericardium).

Left ventricular hypertrophy

In patients who have the electrocardiographic LVH pattern, ST segment/T wave changes are encountered in approximately 70% of cases; these changes result from altered repolarization of the ventricular myocardium caused by LVH [16,19] and are collectively and incorrectly referred to as the strain pattern The electrocardiographic abnormalities seen in this scenario most often involve the ST segment and T wave. ST segment abnormalities (depression and elevation) and T wave changes (prominence or inversion) are encountered. These ST segment/T wave abnormalities are the new norm in many patients who have the electrocardiographic LVH pattern. In a prehospital setting, most chest pain patients manifesting electrocardiographic STE did not have AMI as a final hospital diagnosis; rather, LVH accounted for a significant portion of these patients [6]. The ED population demonstrates a similar trend [7,8]. Furthermore, Larsen and colleagues have shown that the electrocardiographic pattern consistent with LVH is encountered in approximately 10% of adult chest pain patients initially diagnosed in the ED with ACS, of whom only one quarter were found to have ACS. In this study, clinicians frequently attributed the ST segment/T wave changes seen to ACS, when in fact the observed changes resulted from repolarization abnormality associated with LVH pattern [20].

LVH is associated with poor R wave progression and loss of the septal R wave in the right to mid precordial leads, most commonly producing a QS pattern. In general, these QS complexes are located in leads V1 and V2, rarely extending beyond lead V3. STE is encountered in this distribution, together with prominent T waves. The STE seen in this distribution may be

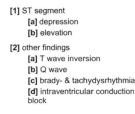

[1] ST segment
   [a] depression
   [b] elevation

[2] other findings
   [a] T wave inversion
   [b] Q wave
   [c] brady- & tachydysrhythmia
   [d] intraventricular conduction
   block

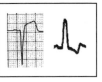

Fig. 8. ECG findings for acute myocarditis.

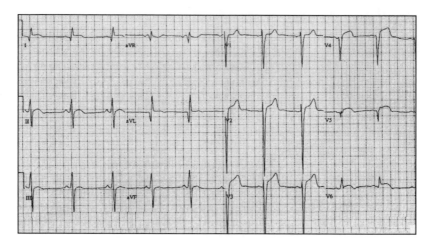

Fig. 9. Acute myocarditis.

greater than 5 mm in height. The initial, upsloping portion of the ST segment/T wave complex is frequently concave in LVH compared with the flattened or convex pattern observed with AMI. This morphologic feature is imperfect; early AMI may reveal such a concave feature (Figs. 10 and 11) [7].

Leftward-oriented leads I, aVL, V5, and V6 frequently demonstrate large, monophasic R waves; these leads typically reveal STD with inverted T waves. This ST segment/T wave complex has been described in the following manner: initially bowed upward (convex upward) followed by a gradual downward sloping into an inverted, asymmetric T wave with an abrupt return to the baseline [21]. The T wave, however, may assume other morphologies, including minimally inverted or inversion greater than 5 mm. These T wave abnormalities also may be encountered in patients lacking prominent

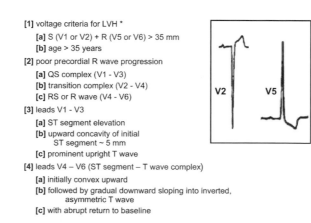

[1] voltage criteria for LVH *
    [a] S (V1 or V2) + R (V5 or V6) > 35 mm
    [b] age > 35 years
[2] poor precordial R wave progression
    [a] QS complex (V1 - V3)
    [b] transition complex (V2 - V4)
    [c] RS or R wave (V4 - V6)
[3] leads V1 - V3
    [a] ST segment elevation
    [b] upward concavity of initial
       ST segment ~ 5 mm
    [c] prominent upright T wave
[4] leads V4 – V6 (ST segment – T wave complex)
    [a] initially convex upward
    [b] followed by gradual downward sloping into inverted,
       asymmetric T wave
    [c] with abrupt return to baseline

Fig. 10. ECG criteria for left ventricular hypertrophy.

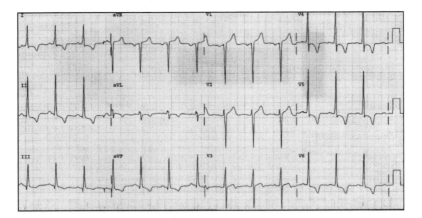

Fig. 11. Left ventricular hypertrophy.

QRS voltage (ie, large S and R waves) typical of LVH [16,19]. Other features of this portion of the ST segment/T wave complex suggestive of LVH-related change include the following: (1) J point depression, (2) T wave asymmetry with rapid return to the baseline, (3) "overshoot" of the terminal T wave at the baseline (terminal positivity), (4) T wave inversions in leads V4, V5, and V6 with the inversion greatest in lead V6, and (5) prominent T wave inversion in lead V6 (greater than 3 mm) (Figs. 10 and 11).

Bundle branch block

Unlike left bundle branch block (LBBB), right bundle branch block (RBBB) does not obscure the electrocardiographic diagnosis of ACS. In BBB, the QRS complex duration is prolonged—greater than 0.12 seconds. Perhaps the most obvious and distinctive electrocardiographic feature in RBBB is a prominent R wave in lead V1. This R wave is broad and may assume any of several morphologies: monophasic R wave, biphasic rSR', or qR formation. In lead V6, a wide RS wave is seen (Figs. 12 and 13).

Significant ST segment/T wave changes are encountered in the patient who has uncomplicated BBB [16]. In general, the correct and appropriate position of the ST segment/T wave complex is dictated by the major, terminal portion of the QRS complex—the rule of appropriate discordance. Using this concept, the ST segment/T wave complex is located on the opposite side of the isoelectric baseline from the major, terminal portion of the QRS complex. As such, leads with predominantly positive QRS complex would present with STD and T wave inversion—discordant STD and T wave inversion. Conversely, a primarily negative QRS complex would be associated with STE and prominent, upright T wave—discordant STE. This concept holds true not only for right and left BBB, but also for VPR, and, to a lesser extent, LVH.

[1] RBBB criteria

    [a] QRS complex > 0.12 sec

    [b] R complex (V1 & V2)

    [c] R, Rs, QS or Qr complex (V5, & V6)

[2] leads V1 – V2 (ST segment – T wave complex)

    [a] depressed ST segment

    [b] inverted T wave

    [c] gradual downward sloping into inverted,
        asymmetric T wave with abrupt
        return to baseline

[3] leads V5, & V6

    [a] variable dependent upon QRS complex configuration

    [b] ST segment – T wave directed opposite of major, terminal portion
        of QRS complex

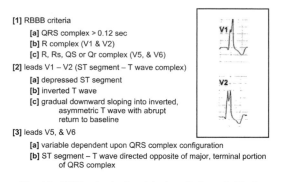

Fig. 12. ECG criteria for right bundle branch block.

LBBB is found commonly among ED chest pain patients, which is unfortunate for several reasons: (1) LBBB is a marker of significant heart disease with extreme risk for acute cardiovascular complication and death in patients who have ACS, (2) LBBB, if new or presumably new and occurring within an appropriate clinical context suggesting AMI, represents an indication for fibrinolysis, and (3) LBBB markedly reduces the diagnostic power of the ECG in the evaluation of potential AMI.

As with RBBB, the rule of appropriate discordance predicts the normal ST segment/T wave findings in LBBB. In the right precordial leads (leads V1 and V2), broad, mainly negative QS or rS complexes are found (Figs. 14 and 15). In these leads, STE with a prominent T wave is seen. The STE in these leads ranges from minimal (1–2 mm) to prominent (>5 mm), although STE >5mm in these leads should spark consideration of AMI [22]. Moving from the right to left precordial leads, poor R wave progression or QS complexes are noted, rarely extending beyond leads V4 or V5. In leads V5 and V6, a positive, monophasic R wave is encountered; the ST segment is depressed in these leads, whereas the T wave is inverted. Similar morphologies are found in leads I and aVL (Figs. 14 and 15).

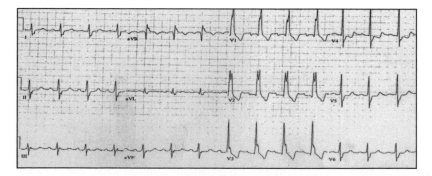

Fig. 13. Right bundle branch block.

[1] LBBB criteria

  [a] QRS complex > 0.12 sec
  [b] QS complex (V1 & V2)
  [c] R or RS complex (I, aVl, V5, & V6)

[2] leads V1 – V2

  [a] ST segment elevation
  [b] upward concavity of initial
    ST segment
  [c] prominent upright T wave

[3] leads I, aVl, V5, & V6 (ST segment –
    T wave complex)

  [a] depressed ST segment
  [b] inverted T wave
  [c] gradual downward sloping into inverted, asymmetric T wave
    with abrupt return to baseline

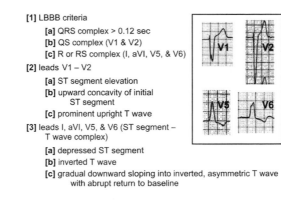

Fig. 14. ECG criteria for left bundle branch block.

Ventricular paced rhythm

As with the LVH and LBBB patterns, right-VPR confounds the ability of the physician to detect ACS on the ECG. Right-VPR not only confounds the electrocardiographic diagnosis of ACS but also imitates ECG findings of acute coronary ischemic events. In right-VPR, the ECG displays a broad, mainly negative QRS complex with a QS configuration in leads V1 to V6; if an R wave is present, it is usually small and does not appear until the left pre-cordial leads, resulting in poor R wave progression. A large monophasic R wave is encountered in leads I and aVL and, on occasion, in leads V5 and V6. QS complexes also may be encountered in the inferior leads (Figs. 16–18).

The anticipated or expected ST segment/T wave configurations are discordant and directed opposite from the terminal portion of the QRS complex—the rule of appropriate discordance—similar to the

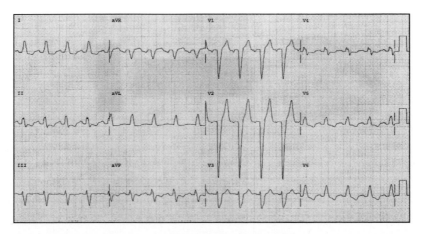

Fig. 15. Left bundle branch block.

[1] right ventricular paced rhythm
    [a] widened QRS complex
    [b] pacer spike in some leads
[2] broad, mainly negative QS or rS complex (V1 to V6)
    [a] ST segment elevation (< 5 mm)
    [b] initial concave morphology
    [c] prominent, upright T wave
[3] monophasic R wave (I & aVL)
    [a] ST segment depression
    [b] inverted T wave

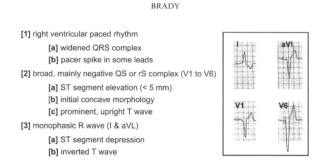

Fig. 16. ECG criteria for right ventricular paced rhythm.

electrocardiographic principles applied to BBB [16,23]. Accordingly, leads with QS complexes demonstrate STE with an upright T wave; this STE is seen in leads II, III, and aVF as well as leads V1 to V6, depending on the positioning of the pacemaker electrode. Leads with a large monophasic R wave demonstrate STD with T wave inversion (Figs. 16–18) [24].

Left ventricular aneurysm

One structural complication of extensive myocardial infarction is ventricular aneurysm, most often arising from the left ventricle after a large transmural infarction. The most frequent electrocardiographic manifestation of ventricular aneurysm is STE (Figs. 19 and 20). Because of the frequent anterior location of ventricular aneurysm, STE is observed most often in leads I, aVl, and V1 to V6. An inferior wall ventricular aneurysm would reveal STE in the inferior leads, though usually less pronounced than that seen with the anterior left ventricular aneurysm. The actual ST segment abnormality may manifest varying morphologies, ranging from obvious, convex STE to minimal, concave elevations.

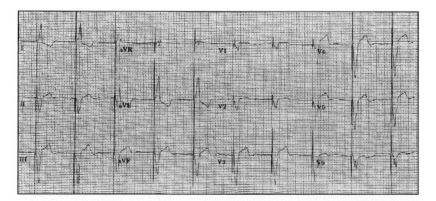

Fig. 17. Right ventricular paced rhythm, with ventricular pacing spikes.

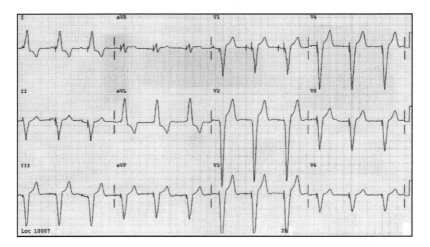

Fig. 18. Right ventricular paced rhythm with atrial and ventricular pacing spikes.

In patients who have ventricular aneurysm, significant Q waves are observed in the same distribution as the STE. The calculation of the ratio of the amplitude of the T wave to that of the QRS complex may help distinguish anterior AMI from ventricular aneurysm. If the ratio of the amplitude of the T wave/QRS complex exceeds 0.36 in any single lead, the ECG likely reflects AMI. If this ratio is less than 0.36 in all leads, however, the findings are likely caused by ventricular aneurysm (Fig. 20) [25].

Other non-ACS causes of ST segment/T wave abnormalities

Cardiomyopathy may produce electrocardiographic patterns that simulate findings associated with acute and chronic coronary syndromes [16]. These findings include significant Q waves, ST segment changes, T wave

[1] past MI
    [a] Q wave
    [b] poor R wave progression
[2] persistent ST segment elevation
    [a] varying magnitudes
    [b] varying morphologies
[3] variable T wave (normal to inverted)
[4] relationship of QRS complex to T wave
    [a] predominant, prominent QRS complex relative to T wave
    [b] T wave / QRS complex amplitude ratio < 0.36

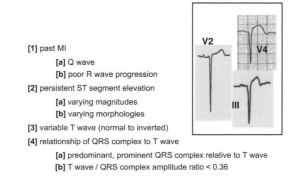

Fig. 19. ECG findings for left ventricular aneurysm.

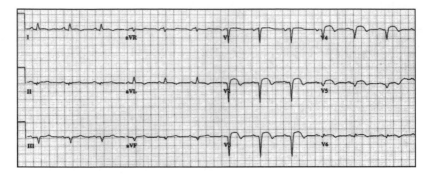

Fig. 20. Left ventricular aneurysm.

abnormalities, and BBB patterns. Cardiomyopathy may produce significant Q waves in the inferior and right precordial distributions; in certain cases, such Q waves may be seen across the precordium, involving the entire anterolateral region of ECG. These leads also can demonstrate STE with prominent T waves. In most instances, the STE is usually less than 5 mm in height with a concave, initial upsloping portion of the ST segment/T wave complex.

In 1992, Pedro and Josep Brugada described a new syndrome that was associated with sudden death in individuals who have a structurally normal heart and no evidence of atherosclerotic coronary disease [26]. Patients who have this syndrome were noted to have a distinct set of electrocardiographic abnormalities, characterized by an RBBB pattern with STE in the right precordial leads. Patients who have this Brugada syndrome have a tendency for sudden cardiac death resulting from polymorphic ventricular tachycardia [27]. ECG abnormalities (Fig. 21) that suggest the diagnosis include RBBB (complete or incomplete) and STE in leads V1, V2, or V3. Two types of STE (Fig. 21) morphologies have been described: convex upwards (coved) and concave upwards (saddle-type) [28–30]. The ECG morphologies may transform from one type to the other or may normalize completely.

[1] RBBB criteria
　　[a] widened QRS complex
　　　　-- incomplete
　　　　-- complete (> 0.12 sec)
　　[b] R or RS complex (V1 & V2)
　　[c] QS or Qr complex (V5 & V6)
[2] ST segment elevation in leads V1, V2, & V3
[3] ST segment morphologies
　　[a] convex ("coved")
　　[b] saddle-type

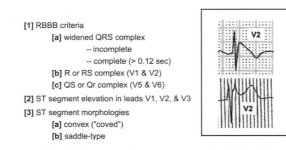

Fig. 21. ECG findings for Brugada syndrome-related ST segment/T wave abnormalities.

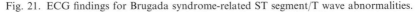

Left ventricular apical ballooning syndrome, also known as Takastubo syndrome, is a recently described disorder in which patients develop anginal symptoms with acute congestive heart failure during times of stress. At cardiac catheterization, these patients are found to have abnormal left ventricular function but normal coronary arteries [31,32]. Classic electrocardiographic findings (Fig. 22) encountered in this syndrome include STE, T wave inversion, and abnormal Q waves [33]. These findings are most often transient, presenting only when the patient is symptomatic and resolving during physiologically normal periods. The STE itself has a similar morphology to that seen in the patient who has AMI [33].

At therapeutic levels, digitalis produces characteristic electrocardiographic changes, referred to as the digitalis effect. The electrocardiographic manifestations (Fig. 23) of digitalis are as follows: (1) "scooped" STD, most prominent in the inferior and precordial leads (those with the largest R wave) and usually absent in the rightward leads; (2) flattened T waves; (3) increased U waves; and (4) shortening of the QT interval.

The earliest sign of hyperkalemia is the appearance of tall, symmetric T waves, described as hyperacute, which may be confused with the hyperacute T wave of early STE AMI. As the serum potassium level increases, the T waves tend to become taller, peaked, and narrowed in a symmetric fashion in the anterior distribution (Fig. 24). Hyperkalemic T waves tend to be tall, narrow, and peaked with a prominent or sharp apex. Also, these T waves tend to be symmetric in morphology (Fig. 24). Conversely, the hyperacute T waves of early AMI are often asymmetric with a broad base. As the serum level continues to increase, the QRS complex widens (Fig. 24), which can make the ST segment seem elevated. This pseudo-STE associated with hyperkalemia is characterized by J point elevation and prominent T waves.

The Wolff Parkinson White syndrome (WPW) frequently presents with evidence of ventricular pre-excitation or actual dysrhythmic events. Such evidence of pre-excitation includes the classic electrocardiographic triad of PR interval shortening, a delta wave, and QRS complex widening. The patient

[1] ST segment elevation

[2] T wave inversion

[3] pathologic Q waves

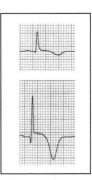

Fig. 22. ECG findings for Takastubo cardiomyopathy.

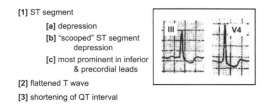

[1] ST segment
  [a] depression
  [b] "scooped" ST segment depression
  [c] most prominent in inferior & precordial leads
[2] flattened T wave
[3] shortening of QT interval

Fig. 23. ECG Findings for digoxin effect.

may present with paroxysmal supraventricular tachycardia that does not reflect the underlying WPW syndrome, rapid, bizarre atrial fibrillation, broad-complex tachycardia, or sudden cardiac death. Various pseudoinfarction findings may be observed that, if not recognized, may once again lead the uninformed clinician to the wrong diagnostic conclusion. Q waves can be seen in leads II, III, and aVF, mimicking past inferior myocardial infarction, and tall R waves in the right precordial leads are suggestive of a posterior wall AMI. T wave inversions can be seen in leads with prominent R waves (Fig. 25).

With the development of hypothermia, the ECG manifests numerous ECG abnormalities, particularly an unusual form of STE (Fig. 26). This hypothermia-related electrocardiographic change involves the juncture between the terminal portion of the QRS complex and the initial ST segment—the J point. The J point itself and the immediately adjacent ST segment seem to have lifted unevenly off the isoelectric baseline, producing the J wave (also know as the Osborn J wave). In general, the amplitude of the J wave is directly proportional to the degree of hypothermia. Other electrocardiographic features associated with hypothermia include (1) bradycardia, (2) tremor artifact, (3) prolongation of the PR and QT intervals, (4) T wave inversions in leads with preeminent J waves, and (5) dysrhythmias such as atrial fibrillation and ventricular fibrillation (Fig. 26).

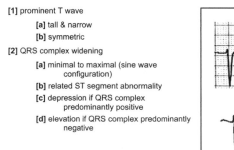
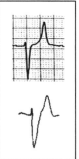

[1] prominent T wave
  [a] tall & narrow
  [b] symmetric
[2] QRS complex widening
  [a] minimal to maximal (sine wave configuration)
  [b] related ST segment abnormality
  [c] depression if QRS complex predominantly positive
  [d] elevation if QRS complex predominantly negative

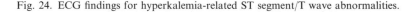

Fig. 24. ECG findings for hyperkalemia-related ST segment/T wave abnormalities.

[1] ventricular pre-excitation syndrome
   [a] shortened PR interval
   [b] delta wave
   [c] widened QRS complex
[2] T wave inversion
[3] ST segment
   [a] depression
   [b] elevation
[4] pathologic Q wave

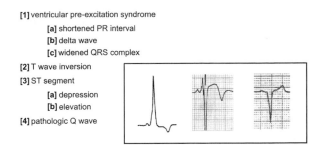

Fig. 25. ECG findings of Wolff-Parkinson-White syndrome-related ST segment/T wave abnormalities.

Central nervous system events such as subarachnoid and intraparenchymal hemorrhage can present with ST segment/T wave abnormalities. These CNS disasters may manifest electrocardiographic abnormality, most often significant T wave inversion in the precordial leads; other electrocardiographic abnormalities such as STD and STE, however, also are seen.

ST segment/T wave abnormalities—electrocardiographic distinction from acute coronary syndrome

If the ECG reveals ST segment or T wave changes (Fig. 27), the clinician then is confronted with the challenge of identifying the source of the electrocardiographic abnormality. In addition to clinical correlation, specific attributes of these ECG findings aid in reaching a diagnosis. QRS complex magnitude (a criterion for LVH pattern diagnosis) and the width (a criterion for BBB or VPR) should be considered first. If either of these abnormalities is present, a confounding electrocardiographic pattern is present, complicating the analysis. Furthermore, the presence of one of these patterns serves to forewarn that ST segment or T wave abnormalities will be encountered;

[1] J wave or Osborn wave
   [a] positive deflection at
      J point
   [b] associated ST segment
      elevation
[2] other findings
   [a] bradydysrhythmia
   [b] muscle tremor artifact

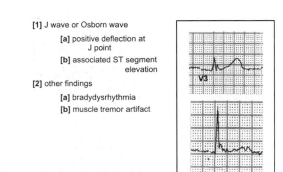

Fig. 26. ECG findings for hypothermia.

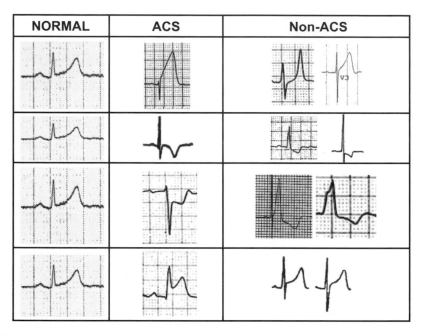

Fig. 27. Specific ECG findings (prominent T wave, T wave inversion, ST segment depression, and ST segment elevation) in normal, ACS, and non-ACS presentations.

these abnormalities can represent the normal findings associated with these patterns or, alternatively, ACS changes superimposed on the confounding pattern.

If a confounding pattern is not seen, the ST segment should be scrutinized, considering the presence of either STE or STD. From the anatomic perspective, the location of the elevation is suggestive of the electrocardiographic diagnosis in two circumstances. First, widespread anterior STE most often is caused by a non-AMI process, including LVH, BBB, and BER [34]. These patterns, when considered as a whole, are encountered much more frequently than AMI occurring in the anterior area [34].

Second and perhaps more important, inferior STE, particularly when isolated, results from AMI in most instances [34]. Again, the most commonly encountered non-infarction causes of STE usually have electrocardiographically widespread or diffuse STE [23,35,36]. Isolated STE is a rare finding in BER [35], whereas isolated STE is not found in LVH and BBB presentations [23,35]. Similarly, lateral wall STE is an electrocardiographic finding more often the result of AMI [34].

The morphology of the elevated ST segment is a predictor of etiology. The use of ST segment waveform analysis has been reported as a useful adjunct in establishing the electrocardiographic diagnosis of AMI [7]. Using this analysis, a concave ST segment pattern is seen significantly more often in the non-AMI patient, whereas the non-concave morphology is seen almost exclusively in the patient who has AMI. As with most guidelines, it is not infallible; patients who have STE caused by AMI may demonstrate concavity of this portion of the waveform.

STD can occur as the sole finding on the ECG or as a component of a more complicated electrocardiographic presentation. If present as the major electrocardiographic abnormality, the morphology of STD is an important consideration. Horizontal (flat) or downsloping ST segment depression is associated more often with ACS, although nonischemic causes of STD also may present with similar morphologies [37]. Reciprocal STD is defined as depression in leads anatomically opposite, or near-opposite, to those with STE (eg, STD in lead aVL in inferior STE AMI). Its presence on the ECG supports the diagnosis of AMI with high sensitivity, and positive predictive values greater than 90%. The use of reciprocal change in prehospital and ED chest pain patients retrospectively increased the diagnostic accuracy in the electrocardiographic recognition of AMI [6]. It is perhaps most useful in patients who have chest pain and STE of questionable cause. The STD occurring in an LVH, BBB, or VPR does not meet criteria for reciprocal ST segment depression.

Considering the magnitude of ST segment changes, the total amount of STE is greater in the patient who has AMI compared with the non-infarction patient. Furthermore, the total quantity of ST segment deviation, ie, the sum of STE and STD, is significantly greater in the patient who has AMI [34].

Summary

The 12-lead ECG furnishes invaluable information in patients who present with chest pain or other symptomatology suggestive of ACS. The ECG can demonstrate abnormalities in a subset of these individuals, ranging from minimal nonspecific ST segment/T wave changes to pronounced STE. The electrocardiographic differential diagnosis of these abnormalities includes not only AMI and ACS, but also BER, myopericarditis, LVH, BBB, VPR, ventricular aneurysm, and other non-ACS entities. A sound review of the 12-lead ECG, together with knowledge of the expected electrocardiographic abnormalities associated with these common diseases, assists the clinician in differentiating ACS and non-ACS ST segment and T wave abnormalities on the 12-lead ECG.

References

[1] Brady WJ, Adams M, Burry SD, et al. The impact of the 12-lead ECG on ED evaluation and management. Acad Emerg Med 2002;40:S47.
[2] Hayden GE, Brady WJ, Perron AD, et al. Electrocardiographic T wave inversion: differential diagnosis in the chest pain patient. Am J Emerg Med 2002;20:252–62.
[3] Somers M, Brady WJ, Perron AD, et al. Prominent T waves: electrocardiographic differential diagnosis. Am J Emerg Med 2002;20:243–51.

[4] Pollen T, Brady WJ, Perron AD. Electrocardiographic ST segment depression. Am J Emerg Med 2001;19:303–9.

[5] Brady WJ, Dobson T, Holstege C, et al. Electrocardiographic ST segment depression: association with ACS. Acad Emerg Med 2004;11:578.

[6] Otto LA, Aufderheide TP. Evaluation of STE criteria for the prehospital electrocardiographic diagnosis of acute myocardial infarction. Ann Emerg Med 1994;23:17–24.

[7] Brady WJ, Syverud SA, Beagle C, et al. Electrocardiographic STE: the diagnosis of AMI by morphologic analysis of the ST segment. Acad Emerg Med 2001;8:961–7.

[8] Brady WJ, Perron AD, Martin ML, et al. Electrocardiographic STE in emergency department chest pain center patients: etiology responsible for the ST segment abnormality. Am J Emerg Med 2001;19:25–8.

[9] Miller DH, Kligfield P, Schreiber TL, et al. Relationship of prior myocardial infarction to false-positive electrocardiographic diagnosis of acute injury in patents with chest pain. Arch Intern Med 1987;147:257–61.

[10] Klatsky AL, Oehm R, Cooper RA, et al. The early repolarization normal variant electrocardiogram: correlates and consequences. Am J Med 2003;115:171–7.

[11] Mehta MC, Jain AC. Early repolarization on scalar electrocardiogram. Am J Med Sci 1995;309:305–11.

[12] Thomas J, Harris E, Lassiter G. Observations on the T wave and S-T segment changes in the precordial electrocardiogram of 320 young Negro adults. Am J Cardiol 1960;5:468–74.

[13] Wasserburger RM, Alt WJ, Lloyd C. The normal RS-T segment elevation variant. Am J Cardiol 1961;8:184–92.

[14] Kabara H, Phillips J. Long-term evaluation of early repolarization syndrome (normal variant RS-T segment elevation). Am J Cardiol 1976;38:157–61.

[15] Hackworthy RA, Vogel MB, Harris PJ. Relationship between changes in ST-segment elevation and patency of the infarct-related coronary artery in acute myocardial infarction. Am Heart J 1986;112:279–88.

[16] Aufderheide TP, Brady WJ. Electrocardiography in the patient with myocardial ischemia or infarction. In: Gibler WB, Aufderheide TP, editors. Emergency cardiac care. 1st edition. St. Louis: Mosby; 1994. p. 169–216.

[17] Spodick DH. Differential diagnosis of the electrocardiogram in early repolarization and acute pericarditis. N Engl J Med 1976;295:523–6.

[18] Glinzton LE, Laks MM. The differential diagnosis of acute pericarditis from the normal variant: new electrocardiographic criteria. Circulation 1982;65:1004–9.

[19] Huwez FU, Pringle SD, Macfarlane FW. Variable patterns of ST-T abnormalities in patients with left ventricular hypertrophy and normal coronary arteries. Br Heart J 1992;67:304–7.

[20] Larsen GC, Griffith JL, Beshansky JR, et al. Electrocardiographic left ventricular hypertrophy in patients with suspected acute cardiac ischemia—its influence on diagnosis, treatment, and short-term prognosis. J Gen Intern Med 1994;9:666–73.

[21] Rykert HE, Hepburn J. Electrocardiographic abnormalities characteristic of certain cases of arterial hypertension. Am Heart J 1935;10:942–54.

[22] Sgarbossa EB, Pinski SL, Barbagelata A, et al. Electrocardiographic diagnosis of evolving acute myocardial infarction in the presence of left bundle branch block. N Engl J Med 1996;334:481–7.

[23] Brady WJ, Aufderheide TP. Left bundle block pattern complicating the evaluation of acute myocardial infarction. Acad Emerg Med 1997;4:56–62.

[24] Kozlowski FH, Brady WJ, Aufderheide TP, et al. The electrocardiographic diagnosis of acute myocardial infarction in patients with ventricular paced rhythms. Acad Emerg Med 1998;5:52–7.

[25] Smith S, Nolan M. Ratio of T amplitude to QRS amplitude best distinguishes acute anterior MI from anterior left ventricular aneurysm. Acad Emerg Med 2003;10:516.

[26] Brugada P, Brugada J. Right bundle branch block, persistent STE and sudden cardiac death: a distinct clinical and electrocardiographic syndrome. J Am Coll Cardiol 1992;20:1391–6.

[27] Brugada P, Brugada R, Brugada J. The Brugada syndrome. Curr Cardiol Rep 2000;2: 507–14.

[28] Alings M, Wilde A. "Brugada" syndrome—clinical data and suggested pathophysiological mechanism. Circulation 1999;99:666–73.

[29] Monroe MH, Littmann L. Two-year case collection of the Brugada syndrome electrocardiogram pattern at a large teaching hospital. Clin Cardiol 2000;23:849–51.

[30] Furuhashi M, Uno K, Tsuchihashi K, et al. Prevalence of asymptomatic STE in right precordial leads with right bundle branch block (Brugada-type ST shift) among the general Japanese population. Heart 2001;86:161–6.

[31] Akashi YJ, Musha H, Nakazawa K, Miyake F. The clinical features of Takotsubo cardiomyopathy. Q J Med 2003;96:563–73.

[32] Ueyma YA. Emotional stress induces transient LV hypocontraction in the rat via activation of cardiac adrenoreceptors. Circ J 2002;66:712–3.

[33] Tsuchihashi K, Ueshima K, Uchida T. For AP-MI. Transient left ventricular apical ballooning without coronary artery stenosis: a novel heart syndrome mimicking AMI. J Am Col Cardiol 2001;38:11–8.

[34] Brady WJ, Perron AD, Ullman EA. STE: a comparison of electrocardiographic features of AMI and non-AMI ECG syndromes. Am J Emerg Med 2002;20:609–12.

[35] Brady WJ. Electrocardiographic left ventricular hypertrophy in chest pain patients: differentiation from acute coronary ischemic events. Am J Emerg Med 1998;16:692–6.

[36] Brady WJ. Benign early repolarization: electrocardiographic manifestations and differentiation from other STE syndromes. Am J Emerg Med 1998;16:592–7.

[37] Chan TC, Brady WJ, Harrigan RA, et al, editors. The ECG in emergency medicine and acute care. St. Louis: Mosby, Inc.; 2004.

ELSEVIER
SAUNDERS

EMERGENCY
MEDICINE
CLINICS OF
NORTH AMERICA

Emerg Med Clin N Am 24 (2006) 113–131

ECG Manifestations: Noncoronary Heart Disease

Dawn Demangone, MD

Emergency Medicine, Temple University School of Medicine, Jones Hall, 10th Floor,
Park Avenue and Ontario Street, Philadelphia, PA 19140, USA

Pericarditis

Pericarditis, or inflammation of the pericardium, is the most common disorder of the pericardium [1]. The list of identified causes is vast. Infectious etiologies include viruses, bacteria, fungi, rickettsia, and parasites, among others [2]. Pericarditis also may manifest following embarrassment of the pericardium (traumatic or iatrogenic), in association with connective tissue disorders, metabolic abnormalities, contiguous structure disorders, neoplasms, metabolic abnormalities, and a myriad of other etiologies [2]. Furthermore, pericarditis sometimes is associated with myocarditis or pericardial effusions [1], which are discussed separately.

Acute pericarditis is probably the most commonly identified phase of the disease process diagnosed in the emergency department. Patients often describe acute onset of a pleuritic type of chest pain, located in the center of the chest, with radiation to the back. Positional influences typically affect the pain, with alleviation on sitting up and leaning forward. On physical examination, a pericardial friction rub may be present, usually detected most readily during exhalation. Also, patients may demonstrate pulsus paradoxus [1].

The ECG patterns in pericarditis follow a typical evolution as the disease progresses from the acute inflammatory phase through resolution. The duration of ECG abnormalities varies with the different etiologies and may persist from 1 week to months [3].

Pericardial inflammation typically causes an associated superficial myocarditis, or epicarditis. This inflammation causes the typical ECG injury current pattern during repolarization—ST segment elevation—seen in acute pericarditis [4]. As the pericardium surrounds the heart, these inflammatory

---

E-mail address: dawnyoon@comcast.net

changes typically involve a large surface area of the heart, resulting in diffuse ECG abnormalities, in contrast to those changes associated with localized insults [4]. Surawicz and Lassiter described ST segment elevation in 90% of patients in their series of 31 patients who had proven pericarditis [5]. The most common pattern involved ST segment elevation in leads I, II, and V5–V6, which was present in 70% of patients. More extensive involvement indicated by additional ST segment elevation in leads III, aVL, aVF, and V3–V4 was not uncommon, however. In addition to ST segment elevation, ST segment depression may be present. Surawicz and Lassiter described ST segment depression in leads aVR and V1 in 64% of patients with pericarditis [5].

Repolarization abnormalities of the atria, reflected in the PR segment, also are identified frequently on ECG in the presence of acute pericarditis. First, a baseline must be identified to analyze the PR segment. The T-P segment should be used, although it may be challenging to identify in the presence of tachycardia or ST segment elevation [3]. The PR segment frequently demonstrates depression in all leads except aVR, which actually may show PR segment elevation. These PR segment changes are seen most readily in leads II, aVR, aVF, and V4–V6 (Fig. 1) [6–8].

Pericarditis may demonstrate T-wave changes on the ECG as the disease process moves beyond the acute phase [1]. Diffuse notched T waves, biphasic T waves, and low-voltage T-wave inversions have been described with evolving pericarditis [3]. Dysrhythmias are uncommon, but when present are usually supraventricular in origin. Interval abnormalities are uncommon in pericarditis [3]. In patients who have known pericarditis, any development of conduction blocks (atrioventricular [AV] or intraventricular) or

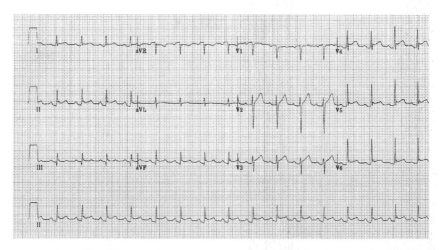

Fig. 1. Pericarditis. A 30-year-old man presenting with pleuritic chest pain. ECG demonstrates many findings associated with acute pericarditis: ST segment elevation most clearly seen in leads I, II, aVF, V3–V6, diffuse PR segment depression, and PR segment elevation in lead aVR.

ventricular arrhythmias is highly suggestive of extension of the disease to myocarditis [3]. Box 1 summarizes the changes seen in acute and evolving pericarditis.

Myocarditis

Myocarditis indicates inflammation of the myocardium, or heart muscle. Most commonly an infectious source is the etiology, with viruses the most frequent causative agent in the United States [9,10]. Myocarditis also may be associated with hypersensitivity reactions, radiation, chemicals, or medications [9].

Clinically the presentation of myocarditis is highly variable, depending on the degree of illness severity. Patients who have myocarditis may be completely asymptomatic, with only transient ECG abnormalities as a clue to their illness [11]. They also may develop a rapid and fulminant disease course leading to dysrhythmias, congestive heart failure, or sudden death [10].

Most commonly the ECG of patients who have myocarditis demonstrates diffuse T-wave inversions without abnormality of the ST segment [3]. When myocarditis and pericarditis occur simultaneously, ST segment abnormalities also may be evident [3]. Rarely patients who have myocarditis demonstrate Q waves, which indicate fulminant disease [3,10].

Myocarditis of any etiology also may affect the conduction system of the heart. The ECG thus may demonstrate QT interval prolongation, incomplete AV block, or intraventricular blocks. Conduction abnormalities are usually transient, and complete AV block is uncommon [3]. Box 2 summarizes the ECG manifestations of myocarditis.

Pericardial effusion and tamponade

Pericardial effusion is defined as an abnormal collection of fluid within the pericardial sac [4]. Pericardial effusion may progress to tamponade,

---

Box 1. ECG manifestations: pericarditis

Acute
Diffuse ST segment elevation, particularly leads I, II, III, aVF, aVL, and V5–V6
Diffuse PR segment depression
PR segment elevation in lead aVR

Evolving
T-wave changes: notched, biphasic, or low-voltage inversions

Box 2. ECG manifestations: myocarditis

Diffuse T-wave inversions without ST segment abnormality
Incomplete atrioventricular conduction blocks (usually
    transient)
Intraventricular conduction blocks (usually transient)

wherein pericardial sac fluid volumes impair ventricular filling [1]. The diagnosis of pericardial effusion and tamponade typically is made by way of echocardiography [1]. The ECG performs poorly as a diagnostic modality for these entities [12]. Two ECG findings classically are associated with these pathologies: low voltage and electrical alternans (Fig. 2). As pericardial effusion and tamponade frequently are associated with pericarditis [1], additional ECG findings consistent with pericarditis also may be evident (see earlier discussion) [13].

The generally accepted ECG requirements for low voltage are: QRS amplitude <0.5 mV (5 mm) in all limb leads and <1.0 mV (10 mm) in the precordial leads [3,12,13]. Kudo and colleagues found that low voltage on the ECG was demonstrated in only 26% of patients who had asymptomatic pericardial effusion [13]. Not surprisingly, the size of the effusion apparently influences the voltage. Studies have shown a higher incidence of low voltage on ECG in individuals who have moderate to large effusions compared with those who have small effusions [12,13]. It is believed that the fluid causes a short circuit effect, resulting in the diminished QRS amplitude [3]. Although low voltage is suggestive of pericardial effusion or tamponade, it

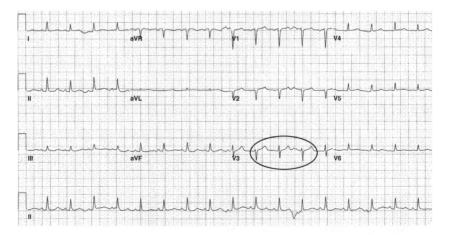

Fig. 2. Pericardial effusion. A 36-year-old man with large pericardial effusion demonstrating evidence of low voltage–QRS voltage <0.5 mV (1 large box) in most limb leads (although not in lead II) and <1.0 mV (2 large boxes) in all precordial leads. Additionally some degree of electrical alternans (phasic morphologic change) is seen in leads II, V2, and V3 (*circle*).

is not pathognomonic, and a large differential diagnosis does exist [3,12]. The P-wave amplitude typically is unaffected by the presence of effusion and tamponade [3].

Electrical alternans occurs in the setting of large pericardial effusions or tamponade [1]. Chou defines it as "cyclic variations in the amplitude of ECG complexes," typically referring to the ventricular complexes displayed on the ECG [3]. Usually the complexes progress between electrical axes over a few cardiac cycles, rather than that of true alternans, which varies from beat to beat. The variability in the complexes occurs as the position of the heart changes during its cycle in a swinging or rotational manner within the fluid-filled pericardial sac (Fig. 3) [3].

Total electrical alternans, an infrequent ECG finding associated with pericardial tamponade, demonstrates cyclic variations in the P, QRS, and T-wave complexes [14,15]. See Box 3 for a summary of ECG findings associated with pericardial effusion and tamponade.

Hypertensive heart disease

Hypertension is a common, typically asymptomatic disease that can be detected and treated easily. The prevalence varies by the definition used and the racial backgrounds of the studied population. The etiology remains unclear in 90%–95% of cases. Left untreated, almost all patients develop increasingly higher levels of blood pressure over time, leading to disease progression and potentially lethal complications [16].

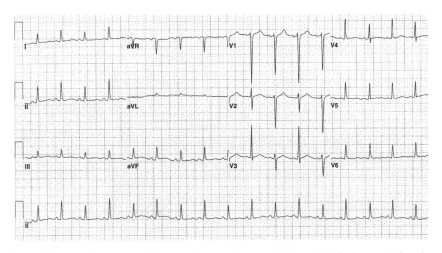

Fig. 3. Electrical alternans. A 36-year-old man with pericardial tamponade demonstrating electrical alternans (best seen in leads V2–V3, but evident in multiple leads, including the lead II rhythm strip).

Box 3. ECG manifestations: pericardial effusion and tamponade

Low voltage
Electrical alternans

In response to the elevated afterload or systemic vascular resistance associated with hypertension, the left ventricle develops an increase in muscle mass, termed left ventricular hypertrophy (LVH). This response is protective only to a certain degree and with time may progress to systolic or diastolic left ventricular dysfunction [17]. Eventually the left ventricle may dilate and function poorly, and the individual develops congestive heart failure [16].

Echocardiography seems superior to the ECG in assessing LVH. Patterns of LVH can show variability by echocardiography. The ECG is unable to discriminate accurately between eccentric hypertrophy, concentric hypertrophy, and left ventricular dilatation [18]. Concentric LVH is associated with higher rates of cardiovascular events and all-cause mortality [17].

The ECG findings associated with LVH may be multiple and can include abnormalities in the QRS complexes and ST segment/T-wave abnormalities (Box 4) [18]. Regionally increased QRS voltage is a frequent finding in LVH. Various LVH criteria exist in the literature, with most centering on the issue of increased QRS voltage. Multiple factors may contribute to this, including an overall increase in left ventricle muscle mass and surface area and a decreased distance between the chest wall and heart [18].

Chou suggests the following as the most commonly used recent voltage criteria to diagnose LVH in patients 40 years or older; these reflect prominent R-wave forces in left-sided leads or prominent S-wave forces in right-sided leads [18]:

S in V1 + R in V6 > 3.5 mV (35 mm)
S in V2 + R in V6 > 4.3 mV (43 mm)
S in V1 > 2.4 mV (24 mm)
R in V6 > 2.8 mV (28 mm)
R in aVL > 1.3 mV (13 mm)

Box 4. ECG manifestations: hypertensive heart disease

Prominent QRS amplitude (left-sided R waves/right-sided
    S waves)
Incomplete left bundle branch block
Intrinsicoid deflection >0.045 sec in leads V5–V6
Left QRS axis deviation
Poor R-wave progression
Q waves right precordial leads or inferiorly

Repolarization abnormalities associated with LVH frequently are termed left ventricular strain. Left ventricular strain represents abnormalities of repolarization (an electrical event), however, and it should not be used as a diagnostic term. In a strain pattern, the ST segment and T wave deviate in a direction opposite that of the QRS complex. In particular, ST segment depression and asymmetric T-wave inversion are evident in leads demonstrating the tallest R waves, typically the left precordial leads, and left-sided limb leads I and aVL [18]. The right precordial leads may demonstrate reciprocal changes, that is, ST segment elevation and prominent T waves [18]. A delay in ventricular depolarization impulse propagation through the increased left ventricular mass and conducting system is believed to contribute to this finding [18]. Other ST segment/T-wave abnormalities, such as flat T waves or slight ST segment depressions in the left precordial leads, also may be present [18]. Presence of these findings in the setting of the increased voltage described lends further support to a diagnosis of LVH (Fig. 4) [18].

An intraventricular conduction delay also may be apparent in LVH, although the overall QRS duration typically remains less than 0.12 sec. Incomplete left bundle branch frequently is identified in the presence of LVH [18]. More specifically, however, the intrinsicoid deflection of the QRS complex may be delayed ≥ 0.045 sec in LVH. This may be most apparent in leads V5–V6. Late activation of the increased muscle mass is believed to contribute to this finding [18].

Other less specific findings are associated with LVH. Left axis deviation beyond $-30°$ may be present but is not sensitive [18]. The right and mid-precordial leads may demonstrate poor R-wave progression, with the equiphasic precordial QRS complex shifting further leftward. Occasionally

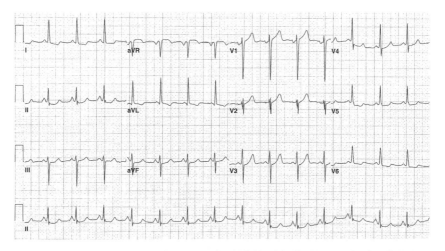

Fig. 4. Left ventricular hypertrophy. A 51-year-old man with ECG findings of LVH (S in V1 >24 mm, R in aVL >13 mm) with strain pattern (ST segment depression and asymmetric T-wave inversions in leads I, aVL, V5, and V6 consistent with repolarization abnormality).

abnormal Q waves inferiorly (most often in leads III and aVF) or QS complexes in the right precordial leads may falsely suggest myocardial infarction [18].

Dextrocardia

Dextrocardia refers to the abnormal positioning of the heart in the right hemithorax. It may or may not occur in association with situs inversus [19], which refers to a mirror image of the organs within the body while maintaining normal anterior–posterior relationships. The atria and ventricles typically are reversed in situs inversus also; thus the heart functions normally [19]. The physical examination may suggest situs inversus with right-sided heart sounds and a left-sided liver [19]. When dextrocardia is not associated with situs inversus, other congenital anomalies are virtually always present, and the condition is apparent before adulthood [20].

The ECG appears somewhat reversed with dextrocardia (Box 5). Lead I is frequently suggestive of the abnormality, with a largely negative QRS complex and inverted P and T waves. Furthermore, the QRS complexes in leads aVR and aVL appear reversed. In the precordial leads, the typical QRS complex progression appears as a mirror image of the normal pattern (Fig. 5) [19]. The precordial leads are helpful when differentiating dextrocardia from right and left arm electrode reversal. When upper limb electrodes are reversed, the ECG demonstrates a normal precordial pattern [20].

Brugada syndrome

In 1992 Brugada and Brugada first described a syndrome in eight patients who experienced aborted sudden cardiac death with structurally normal hearts and similar ECG abnormalities [21]. Patients seemed to have unpredictable, unexplained episodes of polymorphic ventricular tachycardia. Since this initial description, the frequency of syndrome recognition has increased, and it is now believed that Brugada syndrome represents up to 40%–60% of cases of idiopathic ventricular fibrillation [22].

Demonstrated in adults and children, familial clusters were noted in the original report, suggesting a genetic link [21]. A genetic mutation affecting the cardiac sodium channels now has been identified and related to the syndrome [23]. Other factors, including body temperature, certain medications,

---

Box 5. ECG manifestations: dextrocardia

Negative P-QRS-T complex in lead I
Reversed appearance of leads aVR and aVL
Abnormal precordial QRS complex progression

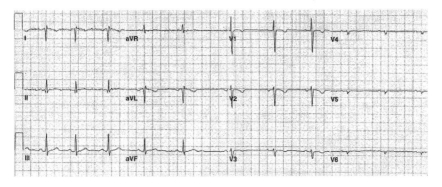

Fig. 5. Dextrocardia. ECG of a 24-year-old woman with dextrocardia associated with situs inversus. Lead I demonstrates negatively directed P-QRS-T complex. Leads aVL and aVR appear reversed. Precordial QRS progression appears mirror image of normal—voltage diminishes as the left precordial leads progress. *Used with permission from* Demangone DA. ECG findings associated with situs inversus. J Emerg Med 2004;27:179–81.

and neurogenic influences, also may affect the predilection for development of ventricular fibrillation in patients who have Brugada syndrome [24].

Individuals may experience self-limited episodes of ventricular tachycardia, resulting in a near-syncopal or syncopal event [24]. If the dysrhythmia continues without intervention, degeneration to ventricular fibrillation can occur, leading to sudden cardiac death [24]. Any patient suspected of having Brugada syndrome must undergo electrophysiologic testing to confirm the diagnosis. Once confirmed, patients are referred for internal cardioverter-defibrillator (ICD) placement [24].

Brugada and Brugada first described the ECG abnormalities associated with this syndrome as consisting of a right bundle branch (RBBB) pattern and ST segment elevation of at least 0.1 mV in leads V1–V3 (Fig. 6) (Box 6) [21]. The ST segment elevation has been described in two morphologies: saddle back, which appears concave upward, and coved, which appears convex upward (Fig. 7) [22,25]. The PR and QT intervals are normal [21]. Although the ECG abnormalities are typically persistent, the ECG may normalize transiently, making the diagnosis difficult [26]. Patients may demonstrate an incomplete RBBB pattern rather than a true RBBB and may have ST segment elevation limited to leads V1–V2 [24].

When Brugada syndrome is suspected, referral for electrophysiologic testing is of the utmost importance, because the mortality rate may be as high as 30% at 2 years without ICD placement [23].

Cardiac transplantation

The ECG following cardiac transplantation may demonstrate various findings, including rhythm and conduction abnormalities; acute transplant

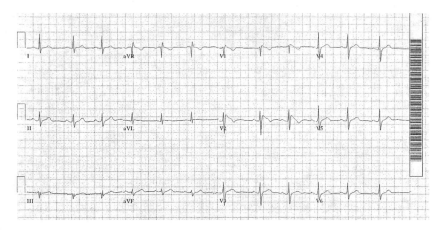

Fig. 6. Brugada syndrome. Incomplete right bundle branch block with ST segment elevation in V1–V2 in the coved pattern. *Used with permission from* Mattu A, Rogers RL, Kim H, et al. The Brugada syndrome. Am J Emerg Med 2003;21:146–51.

rejection also may be reflected on the ECG. Inherent to the procedure is the interesting finding of dual P waves. Retained recipient atrial tissue serves as a site to secure the donor heart, and thus the native and the donor SA node may produce P waves [20]. Typically, native P waves are of smaller amplitude than those of the donor organ [20]. The two SA nodes fire independently, with the donor P waves in synchrony with the QRS complexes (Fig. 8) [27]. Furthermore, the transplanted heart usually contracts at a more rapid rate than the atrial remnant because of surgical autonomic denervation [20,28]. Commonly, native P waves are not detectable because of their small amplitude, the presence of SA dysfunction, or atrial fibrillation before transplant [20].

More than 80% of heart transplant patients demonstrate a complete or incomplete RBBB (Fig. 9). Approximately 7%–25% of patients also demonstrate findings consistent with left anterior fascicular block [20]. Rhythm disturbances following cardiac transplantation include sinus bradycardia, junctional rhythms, atrial tachydysrhythmias, first-degree AV block, and premature ventricular complexes [29–31]. Also, nonspecific ST segment/T-wave abnormalities are fairly common in the postoperative period, likely caused by some degree of pericarditis [20]. Box 7 summarizes the key changes often seen in the ECG after cardiac transplantation.

Box 6. ECG manifestations: Brugada syndrome

Complete or incomplete right bundle branch block
ST segment elevation in leads V1–V3

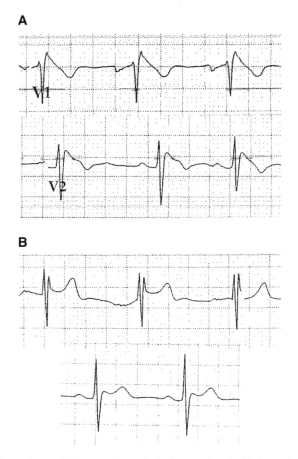

Fig. 7. Brugada syndrome. ST segment morphologies associated with Brugada syndrome. (*A*) Coved appearance with convex-upward morphology. (*B*) Saddle-back appearance with concave-upward morphology. *Used with permission from* Mattu A, Rogers RL, Kim H, et al. The Brugada syndrome. Am J Emerg Med 2003;21:146–51.

Rejection of the transplanted heart may be evidenced by the onset of atrial fibrillation or flutter [32] or prolongation of the QT interval [33,34].

Valvular heart disease

Aortic stenosis

Aortic stenosis (AS) accounts for approximately one quarter of all patients who have chronic, valvular heart disease [35]. It may arise from congenital or acquired lesions, but typically presents as a long, slowly progressive disease of the aortic valve, resulting in increasingly larger degrees of outflow obstruction [36]. The aortic outflow obstruction typically

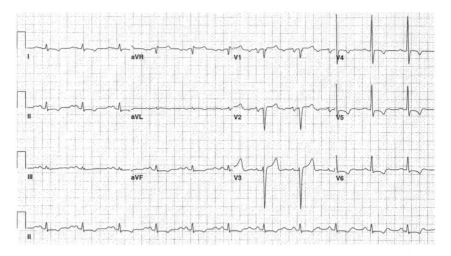

Fig. 8. Cardiac transplantation. ECG of a patient after cardiac transplantation. Dual P waves are visible in the rhythm strip. Note the donor P waves are associated with the QRS complexes, whereas the native Ṕ waves that precede them are not. Thus the Ṕ-P interval is changing; this is best seen in the lead II rhythm strip.

leads to concentric LVH in women and eccentric LVH in men, few may be able to compensate for the obstruction without symptoms for many years [35,36]. Symptoms usually develop in the setting of severe AS, when the valve orifice is only one third the original size [35]. The cardinal symptoms of critical AS include angina pectoris, exertional dyspnea, syncope, and congestive heart failure [36].

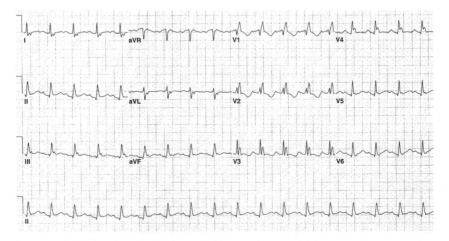

Fig. 9. Cardiac transplantation. Note the right bundle branch block pattern in this patient, a common occurrence (seen in greater than 80%) after transplantation.

Box 7. ECG manifestations: cardiac transplantation

Dual P waves
Faster resting heart rate
Complete or incomplete right bundle branch block

As the normal cardiac response to aortic outflow obstruction is LVH, the ECG typically demonstrates findings consistent with an LVH pattern, with or without strain, (see hypertensive heart disease section) in 85% of patients who have severe AS [36]. Left atrial enlargement also may be apparent in patients who have isolated aortic valve disease, demonstrated by an increased P-wave duration (>0.12 sec) in lead II, or more commonly by a biphasic P wave in lead V1 with a negative terminal portion [36]. Additionally a pseudo-infarction pattern of loss of R waves in the precordial leads is occasionally evident [36].

Rhythm disturbances, such as atrial fibrillation, are not seen commonly. AV and intraventricular conduction abnormalities may be apparent when the conduction system also is affected by calcific changes [36].

Aortic regurgitation

Aortic regurgitation (AR) occurs when the aortic valve leaflets fail to juxtapose effectively during diastole, allowing for the backward flow of blood from the aorta into the left ventricle [35]. Because of the increased volume, the left ventricle typically dilates and hypertrophies. Associated left atrial dilatation and hypertrophy also may occur. Abnormal aortic valve leaflets or an abnormally dilated aortic root can lead to AR; these lesions may be congenital or acquired. Valvular abnormalities most commonly are caused by rheumatic fever [36]. Dilatation of the aortic root may occur with age-related degeneration, cystic medial necrosis (as seen in Marfan syndrome), or multiple other disease processes [36].

Patients who have chronic AR typically remain asymptomatic for several years. By the time patients experience orthopnea, paroxysmal nocturnal dyspnea, or exertional dyspnea, significant myocardial dysfunction has developed. Angina pectoris frequently is experienced late in the disease course [36].

Left axis deviation, or a QRS axis of greater than $-30°$, is typical of chronic AR [36]. Left axis deviation may be recognized easily on ECG by a prominent R wave in lead I, deep S wave in lead III, and a biphasic RS complex in lead II with the amplitude of the S component greater than the amplitude of the R component [37]. LVH with or without a strain pattern is also frequently present [20,36]. Late in the disease course, intraventricular conduction abnormalities may manifest [36].

Mitral stenosis

Mitral stenosis most frequently is the result of rheumatic fever [35], with two thirds of those patients being female [36]. A diminished mitral valve orifice obstructs flow from the left atrium into the left ventricle. Pressures within the left atrium become elevated, and it dilates. As disease progression ensues, pulmonary venous and capillary pressures become elevated, pulmonary compliance decreases, and the patient may develop pulmonary hypertension, eventually leading to right-sided heart failure [35,36].

Typically symptomatic disease develops in the second decade following the rheumatic illness, with functional impairment developing by the fourth decade [35]. Initial symptoms may go unnoticed, because it frequently manifests with exertional activities as dyspnea or cough caused by the acutely elevated pulmonary capillary pressures [35]. As the disease continues, less exertion is required to cause symptoms, and functional disability becomes apparent [35]. Patients also may develop paroxysmal nocturnal dyspnea, pulmonary edema, hemoptysis, pulmonary embolism, pulmonary infections, or infective endocarditis [35].

With mild disease, few changes are apparent on the ECG [36]; characteristic changes are evident in those patients who have moderate to severe disease. Because of the chronically elevated left atrial pressures, left atrial enlargement is evidenced by P-wave duration greater than 0.12 seconds in lead II, or shift of the P-wave axis to between +45° and −30° (Fig. 10) [36]. Additionally the ECG may demonstrate evidence of right ventricular hypertrophy caused by associated pulmonary hypertension. Chou summarizes the principal ECG findings of right ventricular hypertrophy as right axis deviation, tall R waves in the right precordium, deep S waves in the

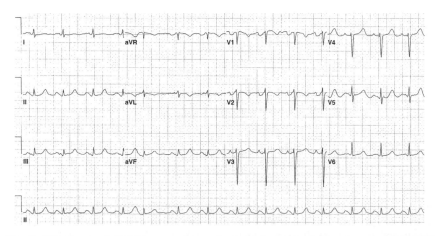

Fig. 10. Mitral stenosis. ECG from a patient who had mitral stenosis demonstrates marked left atrial enlargement; note the broad, bifid P wave in lead II and the large negative deflection of the terminal P wave in lead V1.

left precordium, and a slightly prolonged QRS duration. The unusual electrocardiographic combination of left atrial enlargement and right ventricular hypertrophy thus should trigger consideration of advanced mitral stenosis [18].

Longstanding mitral stenosis frequently is associated with atrial arrhythmias, such as atrial fibrillation or flutter, premature atrial contractions, or tachydysrhythmias, caused by dilatation, fibrosis, and disorganization of muscular architecture of the left atrium [36]. Initial episodes of atrial fibrillation are usually transient, but once permanent atrial fibrillation develops, the disease course progresses more rapidly [35].

Mitral regurgitation

Mitral regurgitation frequently occurs in the setting of congenital abnormalities or rheumatic heart disease [35]. The left ventricle initially attempts to compensate for the increased workload with more complete emptying following systole. As the disease progresses, the left ventricular end diastolic volumes increase and the left ventricle eventually fails. The left atrium also dilates [35].

Most patients who have mitral regurgitation do not experience significant symptomatology. Patients who have more severe disease are likely to describe dyspnea, fatigue, weakness, or orthopnea. And in those who have lowered cardiac output, exhaustion, weight loss, and cachexia may be apparent [35].

The ECG findings associated with mitral regurgitation frequently are nonspecific [20]. With advanced disease, left atrial enlargement and atrial fibrillation are found most commonly [36].

Mitral valve prolapse

Mitral valve prolapse (MVP) may result from various pathologic mechanisms [36] and is present in approximately 2.4% of the general population [38]. It is the most frequent cause of mitral regurgitation. The male to female ratio is approximately 1:2 and it includes all age groups [36]. The syndrome demonstrates significant clinical variability in patients, from the asymptomatic to various nonspecific symptoms to those symptoms associated with significant mitral regurgitation [36].

The ECG in patients who have MVP most commonly is normal in asymptomatic patients. Inverted or biphasic T waves and nonspecific ST segment/T-wave abnormalities in leads II, III, and aVF may be identified in those patients who have symptomatic disease or in a small number of the asymptomatic patient population [36].

Numerous dysrhythmias have been associated with MVP. Premature contractions of the atria or ventricles and supraventricular or ventricular tachydysrhythmias have been reported [39,40]. Patients also may experience bradydysrhythmias or various degrees of AV block. Additionally patients may demonstrate prolonged QT intervals [36]. Box 8 summarizes the electrocardiographic highlights of valvular heart disease.

Long QT syndrome

Long QT syndrome may be of congenital etiology or associated with multiple other causes, such as electrolyte abnormalities, drug toxicities, acute coronary syndrome, central nervous system syndromes, or idiopathic causes [41]. It can be divided into marked or moderate categories. Marked QT prolongation is considered in patients who have corrected QT intervals (QTc) >125% of the normal value; those with moderate prolongation demonstrate QTc values ranging from 115%–125% of the normal values [41]. In calculating the QTc, the generally accepted formula is QTc = QT interval divided by the square root of R-R interval (in seconds). Generally speaking, a QTc <0.44 seconds is considered normal [42].

Box 8. ECG manifestations: selected valvular heart disease

Aortic stenosis
- LVH +/− strain pattern
- Left atrial enlargement
- Pseudoinfarction pattern in precordial leads
- Atrial fibrillation (uncommon)
- AV and/or intraventricular conduction abnormalities (uncommon)

Aortic regurgitation
- Left axis deviation (QRS axis > −30 degrees)
- Left ventricular hypertrophy +/− strain pattern
- Intraventricular conduction abnormalities

Mitral stenosis
- Left atrial enlargement
- Right ventricular hypertrophy
- Atrial arrhythmias

Mitral Regurgitation
- Left atrial enlargement
- Atrial fibrillation

Mitral valve prolapse
- Non specific ST segment/T wave changes
- Tachydysrhythmias
- Bradydysrhythmias/AV block

First described in 1957, congenital long QT syndrome has been genetically linked to abnormalities of the potassium or sodium channels, affecting the ventricular action potential [41]. Congenital long QT syndrome has been associated with sudden death, which often can occur unpredictably or may be precipitated by sudden sympathetic outflow associated with startling stimuli. Patients develop premature ventricular contractions or ventricular tachycardia following the stimuli, which may progress to ventricular fibrillation. The typical pattern of ventricular tachycardia is that of torsades de pointes, which results from a premature ventricular contraction firing during ventricular repolarization or during the T wave. A polymorphic ventricular tachycardia results, with an axis that continues to change direction throughout the dysrhythmia [41].

References

[1] Braunwald E. Pericardial disease. In: Wilson JD, Braunwald E, Isselbacher KJ, et al, editors. Harrison's principles of internal medicine. 12th edition. New York: McGraw-Hill; 1991. p. 981–7.

[2] Spodick DH. Pericardial diseases. In: Braunwald E, Zipes DP, Libby P, editors. Heart disease: a textbook of cardiovascular medicine. 6th edition. Philadelphia: WB Saunders; 2001. p. 1823–76.

[3] Surawicz B, Knilans T. Pericarditis and cardiac surgery. In: Surawicz B, Knilans T, editors. Chou's electrocardiography in clinical practice. Philadelphia: WB Saunders; 2001. p. 239–55.

[4] Goldberger AL. Miscellaneous ECG patterns. In: Clinical electrocardiography: a simplified approach. 6th edition. St. Louis: Mosby; 1999. p. 114–35.

[5] Surawicz B, Lassiter KC. Electrocardiogram in pericarditis. Am J Cardiol 1970;26:471–4.

[6] Spodick DH. The electrocardiogram in acute pericarditis: distributions of morphologic and axial changes in stages. Am J Cardiol 1974;33:470–4.

[7] Spodick DH. Diagnostic electrocardiographic sequences in acute pericarditis: significance of PR segment and PR vector changes. Circulation 1973;48:575–80.

[8] Charles MA, Bensinger TA, Glasser SP. Atrial injury current in pericarditis. Ann Intern Med 1973;131:657–62.

[9] Wynne J, Braunwald E. The cardiomyopathies and myocarditises. In: Wilson JD, Braunwald E, Isselbacher KJ, et al, editors. Harrison's principles of internal medicine. 12th edition. New York: McGraw-Hill; 1991. p. 975–81.

[10] Savoia MC, Oxman MN. Myocarditis and pericarditis. In: Mandell GL, Bennett JE, Dolin R, editors. Principles and practice of infectious diseases. 5th edition. Philadelphia: Harcourt; 2000. p. 925–36.

[11] Wynne J, Braunwald E. The cardiomyopathies and myocarditises. In: Braunwald E, Zipes DP, Libby P, editors. Heart disease: a textbook of cardiovascular medicine. 6th edition. Philadelphia: WB Saunders; 2001. p. 1751–806.

[12] Eisenberg MJ, de Romeral LM, Heidenreich PA, et al. The diagnosis of pericardial effusion and cardiac tamponade by 12 lead ECG. Chest 1996;110:318–24.

[13] Kudo Y, Yamasaki F, Doi T, et al. Clinical significance of low voltage in asymptomatic patients with pericardial effusion free of heart disease. Chest 2003;124:2064–7.

[14] Littman D, Spodick DH. Total electrical alternation in pericardial disease. Circulation 1958; 17:912.

[15] Guberman BA, Fowler NO, Engel PF, et al. Cardiac tamponade in medical patients. Circulation 1981;64(3):633–40.

[16] Williams GH. Hypertensive vascular disease. In: Wilson JD, Braunwald E, Isselbacher KJ, et al, editors. Harrison's principles of internal medicine. 12th edition. New York: McGraw-Hill; 1991. p. 1001–15.

[17] Kaplan NM. Systemic hypertension: mechanisms and diagnosis. In: Braunwald E, Zipes DP, Libby P, editors. Heart disease: a textbook of cardiovascular medicine. 6th edition. Philadelphia: WB Saunders; 2001. p. 941–68.

[18] Surawicz B, Knilans T. Ventricular enlargement. In: Surawicz B, Knilans T, editors. Chou's electrocardiography in clinical practice. Philadelphia: WB Saunders; 2001. p. 44–74.

[19] Marelli AJ. Congenital heart disease in adults. In: Goldman L, Bennett JC, editors. Cecil textbook of medicine. 21st edition. Philadelphia: WB Saunders; 2000. p. 2779–291.

[20] Surawicz B, Knilans T. Diseases of the heart and lungs. In: Surawicz B, Knilans T, editors. Chou's electrocardiography in clinical practice. Philadelphia: WB Saunders; 2001. p. 256–309.

[21] Brugada P, Brugada J. Right bundle branch block, persistent ST segment elevation and sudden cardiac death: a distinct clinical and electrocardiographic syndrome. J Am Coll Cardiol 1992;20:1391–6.

[22] Ailings M, Wilde A. "Brugada" syndrome: clinical data and suggested pathophysiological mechanism. Circulation 1999;99:666–73.

[23] Brugada P, Brugada R, Brugada J. The Brugada syndrome. Curr Cardiol Rep 2000;2: 507–14.

[24] Mattu A, Rogers RL, Kim H, et al. The Brugada syndrome. Am J Emerg Med 2003;21(2): 146–51.

[25] Atarashi H, Ogawa S, Harumi K, et al. Characteristics of patients with right bundle branch block and ST segment elevation in right precordial leads. Am J Cardiol 1996;78: 581–3.

[26] Surawicz B, Knilans T. Acute ischemia: electrocardiographic patterns. In: Surawicz B, Knilans T, editors. Chou's electrocardiography in clinical practice. Philadelphia: WB Saunders; 2001. p. 122–53.

[27] VerNooy RA, Bergin JD. Cardiac transplant. In: Chan TC, Brady WJ, Harrigan RA, et al, editors. ECG in emergency medicine and acute care. Philadelphia: Elsevier Mosby; 2005. p. 223–6.

[28] Alexopoulos D, Yusuf S, Bostock J, et al. Ventricular arrhythmias in long-term survivors of orthotopic and heterotopic cardiac transplantation. Br Heart J 1988;59(6):648–52.

[29] Romhilt DW, Doyle M, Sagar KB, et al. Prevalence and significance of arrhythmias in long-term survivors of cardiac transplantation. Circulation 1982;66(Suppl I):219–22.

[30] Bexton RS, Nathan AW, Hellestrand KF, et al. The electrophysiologic characteristics of the transplanted human heart. Am Heart J 1984;107:1–7.

[31] Locke RJ, Karnik R, McGregor CG, et al. The value of the electrocardiogram in the diagnosis of acute rejection after orthotopic heart transplantation. Transplant Int 1989;2(3): 143–6.

[32] Miniati DN, Robbins RC, Reitz BA. Heart and heart-lung transplantation. In: Braunwald E, Zipes DP, Libby P, editors. Heart disease: a textbook of cardiovascular medicine. 6th edition. Philadelphia: WB Saunders; 2001. p. 615–34.

[33] Ali A, Mehra M, Malik F, et al. Insights into ventricular repolarization abnormalities in cardiac allograft vasculopathy. Am J Cardiol 2001;87(3):367–8.

[34] Richartz BM, Radovancevic B, Bologna MT, et al. Usefulness of the QTc in predicting acute allograft rejection. Thorac Cardiovasc Surg 1998;46(4):217–21.

[35] Braunwald E. Valvular heart disease. In: Wilson JD, Braunwald E, Isselbacher KJ, et al, editors. Harrison's principles of internal medicine. 12th edition. New York: McGraw-Hill; 1991. p. 938–52.

[36] Braunwald E. Valvular heart disease. In: Braunwald E, Zipes DP, Libby P, editors. Heart disease: a textbook of cardiovascular medicine. 6th edition. Philadelphia: WB Saunders; 2001. p. 1643–722.

[37] Goldberger AL. Electrical axis and axis deviation. In: Goldberger AL, editor. Clinical electrocardiography: a simplified approach. 6th edition. St. Louis: Mosby; 1999. p. 44–55.

[38] Freed LA, Levy D, Levine RA, et al. Prevalence and clinical outcome of mitral-valve prolapse. N Engl J Med 1999;341:1.

[39] Kligfield P, Hochreiter C, Niles N, et al. Relation of sudden death in pure mitral regurgitation with and without mitral valve prolapse to repetitive ventricular arrhythmias and right and left ventricular ejection fraction. Am J Cardiol 1987;60(4):397–9.

[40] Stein KM, Borer JS, Hochreiter C, et al. Prognostic value and physiological correlates of heart rate variability in chronic severe mitral regurgitation. Circulation 1993;88(1):127–35.

[41] Surawicz B, Knilans T. QT Interval, U wave abnormalities, and cardiac alternans. In: Surawicz B, Knilans T, editors. Chou's electrocardiography in clinical practice. Philadelphia: WB Saunders; 2001. p. 554–68.

[42] Demangone DA. EKG findings associated with situs inversus. J Emerg Med 2004;27:179–81.

ELSEVIER
SAUNDERS

EMERGENCY
MEDICINE
CLINICS OF
NORTH AMERICA

Emerg Med Clin N Am 24 (2006) 133–143

ECG Manifestations of Selected Extracardiac Diseases

Marc L. Pollack, MD, PhD

Department of Emergency Medicine, York Hospital, 1001 South George Street,
York, PA 17405, USA

Selected extracardiac diseases

The electrocardiogram (ECG) can be altered by various conditions that are external to the heart. Some of these ECG changes are caused by direct cardiac involvement, whereas others result from undetermined mechanisms. These external conditions include physical changes to the heart's position in the thoracic cavity, temperature effects on the heart, abnormal neurologic input to the heart, hormonal abnormalities, increased pressure within the cardiovascular system, or the interposition of fluid or tissues between the heart and the electrodes of the ECG. These ECG findings are often of low sensitivity and specificity in the diagnosis of the noncardiac disease and they may add confusion to arriving at a correct diagnosis. Mimics of acute myocardial infarction (AMI) could, for example, lead to unnecessary thrombolytic therapy with serious consequences. Some ECG findings are helpful in arriving at the correct noncardiac diagnosis. This article focuses on selected extracardiac diseases that cause abnormalities on the ECG of importance to the emergency physician (EP).

Acute pulmonary embolism

Emergency department (ED) diagnosis of acute pulmonary embolism (PE) is difficult and often requires the use of several diagnostic modalities. The patient who has suspected PE often has chest pain and dyspnea, and an ECG invariably is obtained as part of the initial evaluation. The differential diagnosis in these cases often includes acute coronary syndrome (ACS).

E-mail address: mpollack@wellspan.org

0733-8627/06/$ - see front matter © 2005 Elsevier Inc. All rights reserved.
doi:10.1016/j.emc.2005.08.009   *emed.theclinics.com*

Numerous ECG abnormalities have been reported in patients who have PE. Most of these findings have low sensitivity and specificity and are of limited value alone in the diagnosis of PE [1]. The ECG is still useful to the EP, however, when evaluating a patient who has suspected PE. Certain specific ECG abnormalities can make an alternative diagnosis more likely or may be used to assess the severity or prognosis of a PE.

The classic S1Q3T3 pattern first was described in 1935 in a report of seven patients who had acute cor pulmonale secondary to PE [2]. These patients likely had massive PE. Numerous studies over the past several decades have refuted the usefulness of S1Q3T3 [3–5]. Despite having very low sensitivity and specificity for PE, this ECG finding still is often linked to PE. A wide range of additional ECG abnormalities have been described in many published reports over the last 50 years [6]. The problem with many of these published reports is selection bias; many of the study groups included only patients who had massive or large PE.

The exact mechanism of the ECG changes caused by PE is unclear [6]. Large or massive PE causes elevation of pulmonary artery and right ventricular pressures. ECG manifestations are more specific with massive PE [7]. This acute pressure overload on the right side of the heart, acute cor pulmonale, most commonly is caused by PE. This causes right atrial enlargement and right ventricular dilation. This leads to a right ventricular strain pattern and acute right bundle branch block (RBBB) or incomplete RBBB (Fig. 1). In addition, right atrial enlargement manifests as increased height and width of the initial component of the P wave. This is best seen in leads II and V1. Right ventricular enlargement may cause a directional change of the QRS complex waveform from positive to negative in lead I and from predominantly negative to positive in lead V6. Other ECG findings can mimic ACS, such as slight ST segment elevation and shallow T-wave inversion in the inferior leads. In a series of 80 patients who had confirmed PE, precordial T-wave inversion was the most common ECG finding (68%), exceeding sinus tachycardia

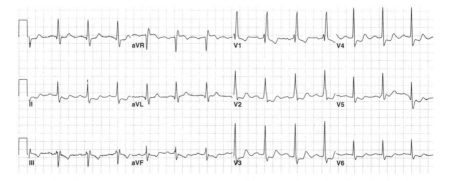

Fig. 1. A 49-year-old woman with acute pulmonary embolism. ECG demonstrates sinus rhythm, RBBB, and ST segment/T-wave changes concerning for myocardial ischemia.

(26%) and S1Q3T3 (50%). Furthermore, the investigators found it to vary with clinical measures of the severity of the PE [8].

Studies have found that in non-massive PE the most common ECG manifestation is normal sinus rhythm [9]. RBBB or incomplete RBBB is a highly variable finding, with a range of 6%–67% [6], and is likely caused by the size and hemodynamic impact of the PE. Other changes associated with PE but lacking sufficient sensitivity or specificity to be helpful to the EP are atrial fibrillation or flutter, sinus tachycardia, axis change, transition zone shift, and ST segment and T-wave changes. A recent observational study examining the usefulness of right-sided chest leads in acute PE found an rS in lead V4R to be sensitive, but the specificity of this finding was not determined [10].

The 12-lead ECG is of limited value in the diagnosis of PE, because there are no ECG findings that are unequivocally diagnostic of PE. The usefulness of the ECG in the patient who has suspected PE is in excluding the diagnosis of other conditions, such as acute MI, cardiac ischemia, and pericarditis. Although the ECG in patients who have massive PE is more specific, the clinical presentation is likely more helpful in arriving at the correct diagnosis.

Pneumothorax

Pneumothorax is a collapse of the lung caused by air in the pleural space. The clinical manifestations vary widely depending on which lung, the percent of lung collapse, the presence of tension, the presence of pre-existing lung disease, and associated injuries or disease. Right and left pneumothorax can produce various changes on the ECG [11–13]. Because these patients invariably present with chest pain, an ECG is usually rapidly available to the EP. ECG findings include decreased QRS complex amplitude, ST segment changes suggestive of cardiac ischemia or infarction, QRS axis deviation, electrical alternans, reduced precordial R-wave voltage, and precordial T-wave inversions. The exact mechanism of these changes is uncertain. Proposed mechanisms include the interposition of air between the heart and the ECG electrodes, interposition of the collapsed lung between the heart and the ECG electrodes, and alteration in cardiac position (especially in tension pneumothorax). Most of these changes resolve with re-expansion of the affected lung. It is important for the EP to realize that ST segment and other changes often found are not necessarily caused by cardiac ischemia.

The extent of the ECG changes correlate with the size of the pneumothorax, whether tension is present, and the side involved [14]. The findings in left pneumothorax include decreased voltage in the precordial leads and QRS axis shift. They comprise most of the cases reported in the medical literature. The ECG findings in right pneumothorax are more ambiguous, less prominent, and less specific but often include reduced QRS voltage and QRS axis changes [11,12].

Pneumothorax cannot be diagnosed by ECG, but perhaps the finding of reduced precordial lead voltage, especially when compared with a prior ECG, prompts a closer look at the chest radiograph. It also is important to remember that pneumothorax can cause ECG changes and that these changes should not be ascribed automatically to cardiac pathology.

Pulmonary hypertension

Pulmonary hypertension (PH) is an elevation of the pressure in the right side of the heart and the final hemodynamic abnormality resulting from many different etiologies. Cases are classified as primary or the more common secondary PH and result in increased right ventricular workload. The final endpoint of untreated pulmonary hypertension is right ventricular failure. The ECG manifestations of the primary disorder causing the PH also are present.

The criterion standard for diagnosis of PH is right-sided heart catheterization, although echocardiography is extremely useful. The diagnosis often is suspected, however, by history and physical examination and careful evaluation of the ECG. In the early stages the disease is difficult to recognize, but the ECG findings may offer a clue. Mild or even moderate PH can exist for many years without becoming clinically evident.

The ECG has a high degree of sensitivity for the detection of abnormalities in symptomatic patients who have PH [15]. Common findings include those that reflect a significant increase over normal in the contribution of the right-sided cardiac structures to the ECG (Fig. 2). As the left ventricular mass normally is three times that of the right ventricle, a doubling or tripling of right ventricular mass is required to pull the electrical forces anteriorly and to the right to produce recognizable ECG changes. The ECG manifestations of right ventricular hypertrophy or enlargement include right axis

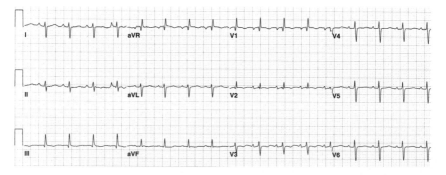

Fig. 2. A 21-year-old woman with pulmonary hypertension. ECG demonstrates rightward deviation of the QRS axis, a qR pattern in lead V1, and S wave > R wave amplitude in lead V6—all consistent with RVH. Echocardiography confirmed the diagnosis.

deviation, incomplete RBBB, prominent R-wave amplitude in lead V1 (R- >S-wave amplitude), qR pattern in lead V1, and rS complexes in the left precordial leads. False patterns of RV hypertrophy can occur in patients who have posterior-wall MI, complete RBBB with LPFB, and Wolff-Parkinson-White syndrome.

Aortic dissection

Aortic dissection (AD) is the most common acute disease of the aorta and it is a diagnosis that should be considered in all patients presenting to the ED with chest pain or back pain. It is caused by blood dissecting into the aortic media after a transverse tear of the aortic intima. Untreated dissection involving the ascending aorta has a 75% 2-week mortality. Timely diagnosis is the key to appropriate management of this condition. Up to 30% of patients who have AD initially are suspected of having other conditions, such as angina, myocardial infarction, or pulmonary embolus. The most common predisposing risk factor is hypertension. Aortic dissection is rare before age 40 years, except in association with Ehlers-Danlos or Marfan syndrome. An ECG is useful in excluding MI but can be misleading in some cases. Thoracic aortic dissections are divided into Stanford types A and B. Type A comprises 62% of patients, involves the ascending aorta, and requires urgent surgical repair. The less common type B often can be managed medically. The DeBakey classification is also widely used and assigns dissections into three types. Type I dissections involve the ascending aorta, the aortic arch, and the descending aorta; type II dissections are confined to the ascending aorta; and type III dissections are confined to the descending aorta (distal to the left subclavian artery) [16,17].

A study from Japan of 89 patients who had acute aortic dissection demonstrated that 55% of the type A dissections had acute ECG changes. These included ST segment depression or elevation and T-wave changes. Only 22% of type B dissections had acute ECG changes, none with ST elevation. The most common complication in type A patients was cardiac tamponade (45%) [18].

The most important use of the ECG is to distinguish acute ST segment elevation MI from AD. Both conditions can coexist, however, when an aortic dissection proceeds retrograde and involves the coronary artery ostium, most commonly the right coronary artery, causing acute proximal coronary artery occlusion [19]. This can produce ST segment elevation in the territory of the occluded coronary artery. Use of thrombolytic therapy in this situation could be associated with an undesirable outcome. Other data (findings on the history and physical examination and the chest radiograph and more advanced imaging of the chest) are critical to aid in the differentiation of these two entities. Fortunately most patients who have AD and ACS have nonspecific ST segment/T-wave changes rather than ST elevation [20].

The incidence of acute aortic dissection erroneously treated with thrombolysis in the European Myocardial Infarction Project was 0.33% (9 of 2750) [21]. As hypertension is common in these patients, the ECG can show left ventricular hypertrophy (Fig. 3). A small study of 43 patients who had aortic dissection found left ventricular hypertrophy to be the most common ECG abnormality (27%) [16]. Dissection also can extend proximally into the atrial septum and atrioventricular (AV) conduction system and cause heart block. In addition, blood can track into the pericardium, causing decreased voltage on the ECG and perhaps hemodynamic compromise.

The EP must be alert to the confounding ECG manifestations that are found in this condition, because the ECG can be normal, show changes associated with longstanding hypertension, or rarely demonstrate changes of acute coronary occlusion.

Central nervous system disease

Acute central nervous system (CNS) events, such as intracranial hemorrhage, trauma, increased intracranial pressure, and nonhemorrhagic strokes, often produce various ECG abnormalities. Conversely, several cardiac conditions can lead to acute CNS events. In some situations, the EP cannot determine which is the primary event. The most common ECG abnormalities are diffuse repolarization abnormalities, such as T-wave changes, ST segment alterations, QT interval prolongation and dispersion, and U-wave changes.

Subarachnoid hemorrhage (SAH) produces ECG changes in up to 80% of patients [22]. The physiologic basis of these abnormalities is controversial but may involve increases in sympathetic and vagal tone that are CNS mediated or actual myocardial necrosis. The most common ECG findings

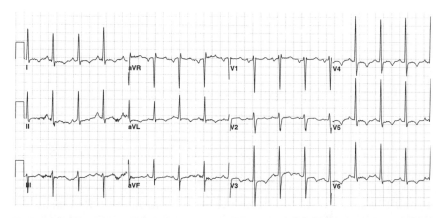

Fig. 3. A 46-year-old man with thoracic aortic dissection. ECG demonstrates sinus rhythm, voltage criteria for left ventricular hypertrophy, and diffuse ST segment/T-wave changes.

include widening and inversion of T waves in the precordial leads, prolonged QT interval, and bradycardia. The EP may be led to suspect a primary cardiac diagnosis, such as acute myocardial infarction or ischemia (Fig. 4). Rhythm disturbances are less common in SAH as shown in a 2002 study of 100 patients who had SAH in whom 93% had a normal sinus rhythm. No significant association was found between mortality in SAH and any single or aggregate ECG abnormalities [23].

Increased intracranial pressure, often associated with intracranial hemorrhage (ICH), produces morphologic ECG changes and rhythm disturbances. Morphologic changes include prominent U waves, ST segment/T-wave changes, notched T waves, and shortening or prolongation of QT intervals [24]. Bradycardia commonly occurs in association with increased intracranial pressure as first described by Cushing at the turn of the last century. A recent study of 50 patients who had ICH demonstrated that increased QT dispersion on the initial ECG is an important prognostic factor [25]. QT dispersion is the difference between the longest and shortest QT intervals on a 12-lead ECG. Increased QT dispersion is associated with an increased risk for arrhythmia [26]. Patients who had brainstem involvement had the largest QT dispersion and the highest mortality but not necessarily from arrhythmias [25]. A case has been published of a patient who had a brainstem hemorrhage, prolonged QT interval, and torsades de pointes [27]. The patient developed T-wave alternans, which is related to ventricular electrical instability and is a marker of vulnerability to ventricular arrhythmias. It is believed that increased catecholamine release is implicated in this process.

Acute ischemic stroke at times is associated with ECG findings of acute myocardial infarction or atrial fibrillation. Patients who have an acute ischemic stroke and an abnormal ECG have significantly higher 6-month mortality when compared with stroke patients who have a normal ECG [28]. Thromboembolic stroke patients often demonstrate prolonged QT intervals, ST segment/T-wave abnormalities, and prominent U waves. In addition, these stroke patients often experience ventricular ectopy.

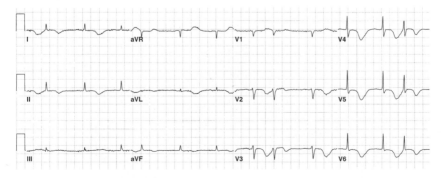
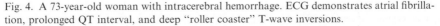

Fig. 4. A 73-year-old woman with intracerebral hemorrhage. ECG demonstrates atrial fibrillation, prolonged QT interval, and deep "roller coaster" T-wave inversions.

Acute CNS events are associated with various ECG abnormalities that have low sensitivity and specificity. ICH is associated with deep T-wave inversion and bradycardia. Findings of acute myocardial infarction or atrial fibrillation are seen in acute nonhemorrhagic stroke; their occurrence may be causative of, rather than resultant from, the stroke.

Pancreatitis, cholecystitis, and other gastrointestinal disorders

Pancreatitis is a serious inflammatory process that is often relapsing, progressive, and may be irreversible; inflammation of the pancreas can affect surrounding tissues. In addition, release of inflammatory mediators can result in a systemic inflammatory response causing multiple organ failure. Another potential complication of pancreatitis is hypocalcemia (Fig. 5). There is significant overlap in the presenting signs and symptoms of acute pancreatitis and ACS. The EP uses the ECG to help differentiate these two entities, but abnormal ECG findings have been reported in patients who have acute pancreatitis [29,30]. The exact mechanism of these changes is uncertain. Postulated causes include a vagally mediated reflex and a direct cardiac toxic effect by pancreatic proteolytic enzymes. No scientific support exists, however, for either of these two proposed mechanisms. Several case reports of patients who have acute pancreatitis demonstrate that findings consistent with ACS, including ST segment elevation, T-wave inversions, and a new left bundle branch block suggestive of acute myocardial infarction can occur [31,32]. These patients had normal cardiac enzymes and normal coronary angiograms. One patient reported on had increased troponins with a normal angiogram, and the investigators suggest a direct toxic effect on the heart by the proteolytic enzymes. A recent study of patients who had alcoholic pancreatitis versus alcoholic and nonalcoholic control subjects demonstrated increased QT dispersion among the pancreatitis patients [33]. The

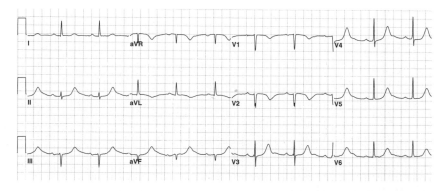

Fig. 5. An 87-year-old woman with acute pancreatitis and hypocalcemia. ECG demonstrates sinus rhythm, prolonged QT interval typical of hypocalcemia, and T-wave abnormalities [8].

investigators in this study, however, did not present sufficient electrolyte data. Hypocalcemia and hypokalemia are associated with a prolonged QT interval.

The ECG is not useful in the diagnosis of acute pancreatitis. The ECG, however, can mislead the EP into an erroneous diagnosis of ACS. The EP must recognize that acute pancreatitis is another cause of ST segment elevation and pancreatic enzymes should be obtained in the right clinical situation. In addition, alcoholic pancreatitis can be another cause of increased QT dispersion. Electrolyte abnormalities associated with pancreatitis can cause ECG abnormalities.

Acute cholecystitis and biliary colic have signs and symptoms similar to those of coronary ischemia. The ECG can have ST segment changes and T-wave inversions. A case series suggests a vagally mediated reflex as a cause of the ECG changes in patients who have cholecystitis or biliary colic [34]. Proper surgical treatment could be delayed while a cardiac etiology is pursued. Once again, this is a cause of a false-positive ECG.

Other acute abdominal disorders can cause nonspecific ECG changes and symptoms suggestive of cardiac disease. A case has been reported of acute gastric distention with retrosternal chest pain and precordial lead T-wave inversions that resolved after nasogastric tube decompression [35]. The mechanism of these reversible changes is unknown.

Sarcoidosis

Sarcoidosis is a systemic granulomatous disease resulting in diffuse fibrotic changes that cause end-organ damage. The etiology is unknown, and virtually every organ can be involved, with pulmonary involvement in 90% of patients. Cardiac sarcoid is more common than previously recognized and likely is present in 27% of sarcoid patients [36]. Patients who have cardiac involvement have a higher mortality. In myocardial sarcoidosis, various portions of the heart wall are replaced by granulomas. Pericardial involvement is much less likely. Because of varied involvement of the myocardium the manifestations are diverse. ECG abnormalities include varying degrees of AV block, bundle branch block, and ventricular arrhythmias [37]. Sudden death has been known to occur, presumably of cardiac origin. Only 20% of sarcoidosis patients manifest signs and symptoms of cardiac involvement. Therapy with steroids may halt progression of left ventricular dysfunction, whereas arrhythmias warrant implantation of a cardioverter-defibrillator device.

Moreover, ECG abnormalities develop in sarcoidosis patients as a result of their pulmonary disease. Almost all patients who have pulmonary sarcoidosis develop pulmonary fibrosis and ultimately cor pulmonale. ECG findings include right heart strain, right ventricular hypertrophy, right bundle branch block, and right atrial enlargement.

The sarcoidosis patient who has pulmonary involvement displays a wide range of ECG findings depending on whether there is coexisting cardiac involvement and on the extent of the pulmonary disease.

References

[1] Stein PD, Terrin ML, Hales CA, et al. Clinical, laboratory, roentgenographic, and electrocardiographic findings in patients with acute pulmonary embolism and no pre-existing cardiac or pulmonary disease. Chest 1991;100:598–603.
[2] McGinn S, White PD. Acute cor pulmonale resulting from pulmonary embolism. JAMA 1935;104:1473–80.
[3] Rodger M, Makropoulos D, Turek M, et al. Diagnostic value of the electrocardiogram in suspected pulmonary embolism. Am J Cardiol 2000;86:807–9, A10.
[4] Stein PD, Dalen JE, McIntyre KM, et al. The electrocardiogram in acute pulmonary embolism. Prog Cardiovasc Dis 1975;17:247–57.
[5] Richman PB, Loutfi H, Lester SJ, et al. Electrocardiographic findings in emergency department patients with pulmonary embolism. J Emerg Med 2004;27:121–6.
[6] Chan TC, Vilke GM, Pollack M, et al. Electrocardiographic manifestations: pulmonary embolism. J Emerg Med 2001;21:263–70.
[7] Petrov DB. Appearance of right bundle branch block in electrocardiograms of patients with pulmonary embolism as a marker for obstruction of the main pulmonary trunk. J Electrocardiol 2001;34:185–8.
[8] Ferrari E, Imbert A, Chevalier T, et al. The ECG in pulmonary embolism. Predictive value of negative T waves in the precordial leads—80 case reports. Chest 1997;111:537–43.
[9] Sreeram N, Cheriex EC, Smeets JL, et al. Value of the 12-lead electrocardiogram at hospital admission in the diagnosis of pulmonary embolism. Am J Cardiol 1994;73:298–303.
[10] Akula R, Hasan SP, Alhassen M, et al. Right-sided EKG in pulmonary embolism. J Natl Med Assoc 2003;95:714–7.
[11] Alikhan M, Biddison JH. Electrocardiographic changes with right-sided pneumothorax. South Med J 1998;91:677–80.
[12] Harrigan RA, McNeil BK. Pneumothorax. In: Chan TC, Brady W, Harrigan R, Ornato J, Rosen P, editors. ECG in emergency medicine and acute care. Philadelphia: Elsevier Mosby; 2005. p. 300–2.
[13] Ortega-Carnicer J, Ruiz-Lorenzo F, Zarca MA, et al. Electrocardiographic changes in occult pneumothorax. Resuscitation 2002;52:306–7.
[14] Strizik B, Forman R. New ECG changes associated with a tension pneumothorax: a case report. Chest 1999;115:1742–4.
[15] Bossone E, Butera G, Bodini BD, et al. The interpretation of the electrocardiogram in patients with pulmonary hypertension: the need for clinical correlation. Ital Heart J 2003;4: 850–4.
[16] Sullivan PR, Wolfson AB, Leckey RD, et al. Diagnosis of acute thoracic aortic dissection in the emergency department. Am J Emerg Med 2000;18:46–50.
[17] Chen K, Varon J, Wenker OC, et al. Acute thoracic aortic dissection: the basics. J Emerg Med 1997;15:859–67.
[18] Hirata K, Kyushima M, Asato H. Electrocardiographic abnormalities in patients with acute aortic dissection. Am J Cardiol 1995;76:1207–12.
[19] Ohtani N, Kiyokawa K, Asada H, et al. Stanford type A acute dissection developing acute myocardial infarction. Jpn J Thorac Cardiovasc Surg 2000;48:69–72.
[20] Kamp TJ, Goldschmidt-Clermont PJ, Brinker JA, et al. Myocardial infarction, aortic dissection, and thrombolytic therapy. Am Heart J 1994;128:1234–7.

[21] The European Myocardial Infarction Project Group. Prehospital thrombolytic therapy in patients with suspected acute myocardial infarction. N Engl J Med 1993;329:383–9.

[22] Perron AD, Brady WJ. Electrocardiographic manifestations of CNS events. Am J Emerg Med 2000;18:715–20.

[23] Sommargren CE, Zaroff JG, Banki N, et al. Electrocardiographic repolarization abnormalities in subarachnoid hemorrhage. J Electrocardiol 2002;35(Suppl):257–62.

[24] Jachuck SJ, Ramani PS, Clark F, et al. Electrocardiographic abnormalities associated with raised intracranial pressure. BMJ 1975;1:242–4.

[25] Huang CH, Chen WJ, Chang WT, et al. QTc dispersion as a prognostic factor in intracerebral hemorrhage. Am J Emerg Med 2004;22:141–4.

[26] Day CP, McComb JM, Campbell RW. QT dispersion: an indication of arrhythmia risk in patients with long QT intervals. Br Heart J 1990;63:342–4.

[27] Chao CL, Chen WJ, Wu CC, et al. Torsade de pointes and T wave alternans in a patient with brainstem hemorrhage. Int J Cardiol 1995;51:199–201.

[28] Bozluolcay M, Ince B, Celik Y, et al. Electrocardiographic findings and prognosis in ischemic stroke. Neurol India 2003;51:500–2.

[29] Khairy P, Marsolais P. Pancreatitis with electrocardiographic changes mimicking acute myocardial infarction. Can J Gastroenterol 2001;15:522–6.

[30] Albrecht CA, Laws FA. ST segment elevation pattern of acute myocardial infarction induced by acute pancreatitis. Cardiol Rev 2003;11:147–51.

[31] Yu AC, Riegert-Johnson DL. A case of acute pancreatitis presenting with electrocardiographic signs of acute myocardial infarction. Pancreatol 2003;3:515–7.

[32] Patel J, Movahed A, Reeves WC. Electrocardiographic and segmental wall motion abnormalities in pancreatitis mimicking myocardial infarction. Clin Cardiol 1994;17:505–9.

[33] Sakagami J, Kataoka K, Sogame Y, et al. Increased QT dispersion in patients with alcoholic pancreatitis. Pancreas 2004;28:380–6.

[34] Krasna MJ, Flancbaum L. Electrocardiographic changes in cardiac patients with acute gallbladder disease. Am Surg 1986;52:541–3.

[35] Frais MA, Rodgers K. Dramatic electrocardiographic T wave changes associated with gastric dilatation. Chest 1990;98:489–90.

[36] Shammas RL, Movahed A. Sarcoidosis of the heart. Clin Cardiol 1993;16:462–72.

[37] Syed J, Myers R. Sarcoid heart disease. Can J Cardiol 2004;20:89–93.

ELSEVIER
SAUNDERS

EMERGENCY
MEDICINE
CLINICS OF
NORTH AMERICA

Emerg Med Clin N Am 24 (2006) 145–157

ECG Manifestations of Selected Metabolic and Endocrine Disorders

David A. Wald, DO

*Department of Emergency Medicine, Temple University Hospital, 3401 North Broad Street,
Jones Hall, 10th Floor, Philadelphia, PA 19140, USA*

Hypercalcemia

Hypercalcemia shortens the plateau phase (phase 2) of the cardiac action potential and decreases the effective refractory period, resulting in shortening of the ST segment [1–3]. Classically this is manifested on the ECG as a shortened QT interval. The QT interval is the distance measured from the beginning of the QRS complex to the end of the T wave [4]. This interval approximates the duration of ventricular systole. The correlation between the duration of the QT interval and the serum calcium level, however, is not linear. It may be unpredictable because of the many factors that affect the QT interval, including: patient age, heart rate, gender, antidysrhythmic medication, and other electrolytes [3]. Because the QT interval varies with cycle length, the rate corrected QT interval (QTc) often is measured to correct for heart rate. The QTc interval is determined by the formula: QT interval/$\sqrt{RR}$. The upper limit of the QTc is, conservatively, roughly 0.44 seconds for both genders, although the normal QTc range in women is slightly longer than in men. Shortening of the QaT interval also is noted in patients who have hypercalcemia. The QaT interval is measured from the beginning of the QRS complex to the apex of the T wave. This occurs because hypercalcemia commonly is associated with early peaking and a gradual down slope of the descending limb of the T wave [4]. The QaT interval correlates best with the serum calcium level [3].

In cases of severe hypercalcemia (serum calcium > 16 mg/dL), the duration of the T wave can increase. When this occurs, the QT interval may seem normal even though the ST segment remains shortened [5–7]. Other ECG abnormalities that may occur in patients who have severe hypercalcemia

E-mail address: waldda@tuhs.temple.edu

0733-8627/06/$ - see front matter © 2005 Elsevier Inc. All rights reserved.
doi:10.1016/j.emc.2005.08.010

include an increased amplitude of the QRS complex, ST segment elevation, diphasic T waves, prominent U waves, and J (Osborn) waves (Fig. 1) [3,4,8].

Hypocalcemia

Hypocalcemia prolongs the duration of the plateau phase (phase 2) of the cardiac action potential [1,4]. Characteristic ECG manifestations of hypocalcemia are prolongation of the QT interval as a result of lengthening of the ST segment (Fig. 2) [7]. Although variable, QT interval prolongation is proportional to the degree of hypocalcemia. When prolonged, the QTc rarely exceeds 140% of normal [9]. When the QTc seems to be prolonged greater than 140% of normal, it suggests that the U wave has been incorporated into the T wave and that the QU interval is being measured.

T-wave changes are not common, because hypocalcemia does not affect phase 3 of the action potential. Decreased T-wave voltage, T-wave flattening, terminal T-wave inversion, or deeply inverted T waves, however, have been described in cases of severe hypocalcemia [4,9,10].

Although rarely reported, hypocalcemia also can be associated with ST segment elevation, mimicking an acute myocardial infarction or T-wave abnormalities simulating myocardial ischemia [9,11]. Coronary artery spasm in the presence of hypocalcemia may play a role in manifesting these ECG abnormalities. Concomitant hypomagnesemia can exacerbate the ECG manifestations of hypocalcemia.

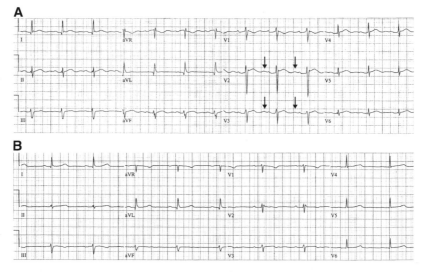

Fig. 1. (*A*) Hypercalcemia. This ECG is from a patient with a serum calcium level of 14.7 mg/dL, demonstrating a shortened QT interval. In addition, prominent U waves (*arrows*) are seen best in the right precordial leads. (*B*) Normocalcemia. This is baseline ECG from the same patient as in (*A*) when her serum calcium level was normalized (7.8 mg/dL). The QT interval is no longer shortened and the U waves are much less prominent.

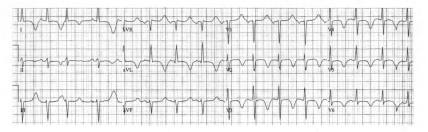

Fig. 2. Hypocalcemia. This ECG is from a patient with a serum calcium level of 4.9 mg/dL. Of note is the prolonged QT interval. The deeply inverted T waves were present on the baseline ECG.

Hyperkalemia

Hyperkalemia initially causes an acceleration of the terminal phase of ventricular repolarization [12,13]. This is responsible for the earliest ECG manifestation of hyperkalemia. As the serum potassium concentration exceeds 5.5 mEq/L, the T waves often become tall, narrow, and peaked (Fig. 3) [9,12–14]. Inverted T waves in the lateral precordial leads usually associated with left ventricular hypertrophy (LVH) can become upright (pseudonormalize) in the presence of hyperkalemia [15]. T-wave changes are usually evident before any change in the QRS complex occurs. Because of variation between individuals and the numerous etiologies of T-wave

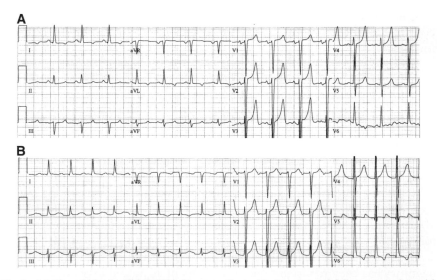

Fig. 3. (A) Hyperkalemia. This ECG is from a patient with chronic renal failure presenting with a serum potassium level of 5.8 mEq/L. Tall, narrow, and peaked T waves are most evident in the precordial leads. (B) Resolving hyperkalemia. This is the baseline ECG from the patient in (A). The ECG was obtained when the patient had a serum potassium level of 4.2 mEq/L. The T-wave abnormalities are no longer present.

abnormalities (eg, bradycardia, cerebrovascular accident, left ventricular diastolic overload, subendocardial ischemia), the ECG diagnosis of hyperkalemia cannot always be made with certainty based on T-wave changes alone [9]. A correct ECG diagnosis of hyperkalemia, however, usually can be made when the serum potassium concentration exceeds 6.7 mEq/L [14].

Hyperkalemia causes a progressive decrease in the resting cardiac membrane potential, which leads to a decrease in the maximum velocity of depolarization (Vmax). A reduction in the atrial and ventricular transmembrane potentials causes a reduced influx of sodium, leading to a decrease in the cellular action potential [13,16]. This results in shortening of the action potential and slowing of intraatrial and intraventricular conduction. Because atrial myocardial tissue is more sensitive to the effects of elevated serum potassium, P-wave flattening and PR interval prolongation may be seen before widening of the QRS complex occurs [13]. When the serum potassium concentration exceeds 7.0 mEq/L, the P-wave amplitude often decreases and the duration of the P wave increases [14]. As the serum potassium level continues to increase (usually greater than 8 mEq/L), the P waves eventually disappear. Progressive hyperkalemia can lead to suppression of sinoatrial and atrioventricular conduction, resulting in a sinoventricular rhythm. Sinoatrial and atrioventricular conduction blocks that often are associated with escape beats also may occur [13]. Accessory bypass tracts are also more sensitive to the effects of hyperkalemia than normal conduction pathways. This can lead to normalization of the ECG and loss of the delta wave in patients who have Wolff Parkinson White syndrome [13].

QRS complex changes are usually evident when the serum potassium concentration exceeds 6.5 mEq/L (Fig. 4). Hyperkalemia generally causes uniform widening of the QRS complex. This widening associated with hyperkalemia affects the initial and terminal portions of the QRS complex. The morphology of the QRS complex often differs from the ECG pattern of a bundle branch block or ventricular pre-excitation. Typically the wide S wave in the left precordial leads can help differentiate the pattern of hyperkalemia from that of a left bundle branch block, whereas the wide initial portion of the QRS complex may help differentiate the pattern of hyperkalemia from that of a typical right bundle branch block [14]. In some cases, however, the wide QRS complex may resemble a pattern of a typical right or left bundle branch block. As the serum potassium concentration further increases, the QRS complex widens progressively. These electrocardiographic abnormalities can be further potentiated by hyponatremia and hypocalcemia [16].

Although uncommon, ST segment elevation simulating an acute current of injury has been reported to occur in cases of advanced hyperkalemia [17–20]. In these cases, a pseudoinfarction pattern may at times represent a diagnostic dilemma for the emergency physician faced with an ECG suggestive of an acute coronary syndrome. These findings can occur in patients who have renal failure and diabetic ketoacidosis. Although the true mechanism

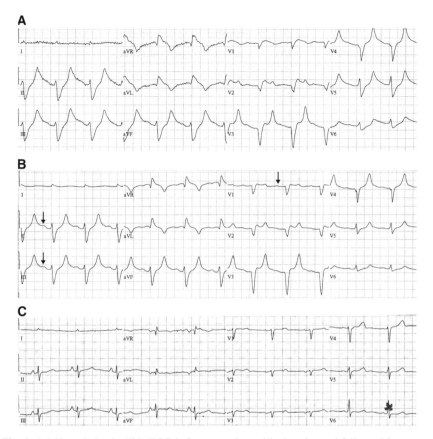

Fig. 4. (*A*) Hyperkalemia. This ECG is from a patient with chronic renal failure with a serum potassium level of 7.7 mEq/L. Note the uniform widening of the QRS complex consistent with an accelerated idioventricular rhythm. P waves cannot be definitely identified. (*B*) Hyperkalemia after treatment with calcium salts. This ECG is from the same patient as in (*A*) after administration of intravenous calcium gluconate. P waves are now barely visible (*arrows*) and the QRS duration has become less wide. (*C*) Normokalemia. This is the baseline ECG from the patient in (*A*) and (*B*). The ECG was obtained when the patient had a serum potassium level of 4.9 mEq/L.

is unknown, it is believed that the ST segment elevation may be caused by nonhomogeneous depolarization in different portions of the myocardium [14].

When the serum potassium concentration exceeds 10 mEq/L the ventricular rhythm may become irregular as a result of activity of different escape pacemaker sites in the depressed myocardium. Above this level, ventricular depolarization is exceedingly slow, and portions of the ventricular myocardium undergo repolarization before depolarization is completed. When this occurs, it may be impossible to determine the end of the QRS complex [14]. As the QRS complex continues to widen, it may blend with the T wave, creating a sine wave appearance. This classically described rhythm is a pre-terminal manifestation of hyperkalemia (Fig. 5). When the serum potassium concentration is greater than 12–14 mEq/L, ventricular asystole or ventricular fibrillation may be seen. Rarely, wide complex tachycardia may occur in the presence of less severe cases of hyperkalemia [14].

The ECG has long been used as a surrogate marker for clinically significant hyperkalemia. Albeit rare, some patients may only exhibit minor ECG abnormalities even in the face of severely elevated potassium [21]. Other electrolyte abnormalities such as hypernatremia and hypercalcemia in addition to metabolic alkalosis may diminish some of the ECG manifestations of hyperkalemia [13]. Although there is usually a predictable correlation between ECG manifestations and severe hyperkalemia, significant individual variations exist (Fig. 6).

Hypokalemia

Hypokalemia increases the resting cardiac membrane potential and increases the duration of the action potential and the duration of the refractory period [4,7]. The characteristic ECG abnormalities associated with moderate to severe hypokalemia include the triad of decreased T-wave amplitude, depression of the ST segment (0.5 mm or greater), and the appearance of U waves (amplitude greater than 1 mm and amplitude greater than the T wave in the same lead) [3,4,7,9,12,22]. These typical ECG findings of hypokalemia are present in approximately 80% of cases when the serum potassium concentration is less than 2.7 mEq/L [9]. These findings, however, are present in only approximately 10% of cases when the serum potassium level is between 3.0 and 3.5 mEq/L. A decrease in the T-wave amplitude occurs first, followed by ST segment depression as the serum potassium level further decreases [13].

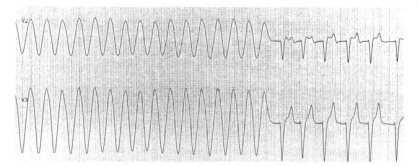

Fig. 5. Sine wave rhythm of hyperkalemia. This rhythm strip is from a patient presenting with a serum potassium level of 8.7 mEq/L. The rhythm strip demonstrates the classic sine wave seen in advanced hyperkalemia. The patient was administered intravenous calcium gluconate, causing an immediate narrowing of the QRS complex.

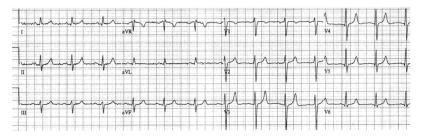

Fig. 6. Hyperkalemia. This ECG is from a patient with a serum potassium level of 6.7 mEq/L. The ECG demonstrates minimal narrowed peaking of the T waves. The QRS complex is normal in duration.

Prominent U waves often are noted in moderate to severe hypokalemia (Fig. 7). Although the origin of U waves is still uncertain, they usually appear as small positive deflections after the T wave and are best seen in the right precordial leads, especially V2 and V3 [9,12]. As long as the T and U waves are separated by a distinct notch, the QT interval can be measured accurately and should remain normal. In severe cases, the T and U waves can fuse to form a single upward deflection. When this occurs, the QT interval may seem to be prolonged. As is often the case, the U wave is included in the measurement of the QT interval, actually representing the QU interval [7,12,23–26]. Because the height (voltage) of the U wave is usually the lowest in lead aVL, this lead should be used to best determine the true QT interval [9].

In severe hypokalemia (<2.5 mEq/L), giant U waves have been described that can be mistaken for peaked T waves similar to those noted in patients who have hyperkalemia [12]. Severe hypokalemia also has been associated with the development of ventricular dysrhythmias, including ventricular tachycardia, ventricular fibrillation, and torsades de pointes in patients without underlying heart disease [14,22]. Concomitant hypomagnesemia may further predispose a patient to developing ventricular dysrhythmias [7].

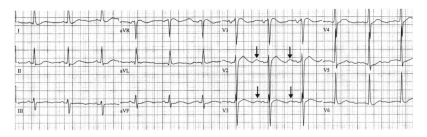

Fig. 7. Hypokalemia. This ECG is from a patient with a serum potassium level of 1.9 mEq/L, demonstrating T-wave flattening and prominent U waves (*arrows*) seen best in the right precordial leads.

Other ECG findings that have been described in patients who have hypo-kalemia include an increased P-wave amplitude and duration and PR interval prolongation [4,9]. In more severe cases, the QRS complex has been noted to widen uniformly together with ST segment depression and T-wave inversion [4]. In adults, the QRS duration rarely increases by more than 0.02 seconds, but this may be more pronounced in children [9].

ECG manifestations of hypokalemia may be difficult to recognize in the presence of sinus tachycardia. This occurs because ST segment depression and decreased T- and U-wave amplitude are common ECG findings in tachycardia [9]. In addition, as the heart rate increases the U wave usually merges with the terminal portion of the preceding T wave and the takeoff of the P wave. This can lead to the appearance of PR segment depression, because the P wave takeoff is above the ECG baseline. This finding usually resolves after correction of the hypokalemia [9]. In the presence of LVH, hypokalemia and coronary ischemia may be suspected when ST segment depression is noted in the right precordial leads. In the presence of uncomplicated LVH, the ST segment usually is elevated in these leads [9].

Hypokalemia also has been associated with various atrial dysrhythmias, including paroxysmal atrial tachycardia, multifocal atrial tachycardia, atrial fibrillation, and atrial flutter [7]. The occurrence of these dysrhythmias may be attributed to an increase in the automaticity of ectopic pacemakers that can occur with hypokalemia [14].

In patients who have an acute myocardial infarction, the presence of hypokalemia has been independently associated with an increased incidence of ventricular dysrhythmias [27–30]. It is for this reason that patients presenting with an acute coronary syndrome should have a prompt evaluation for the presence of hypokalemia and proper correction if needed.

Hypothermia

Hypothermia is defined as a core body temperature less than 35°C (95°F). When this condition occurs certain characteristic ECG findings may be seen. These abnormalities include tremor artifact, slowing of the sinus rate leading to bradycardia, conduction disturbances leading to prolongation of the PR and QT intervals, and the appearance of the classic Osborn or J wave [2,7,31].

Tremor artifact is one of the earliest, although nonspecific, ECG findings in patients who have hypothermia (Fig. 8). The body's ability to shiver diminishes as the core temperature decreases, and is uncommon when the body temperature falls to less than 32°C (90 F) [7]. Sinus rhythm predominates in cases of mild hypothermia.

The Osborn or J wave, also known as the camel-hump sign, is an extra deflection noted on the ECG at the terminal junction of the QRS complex and the beginning of the ST segment takeoff (Fig. 9) [31,32]. The Osborn

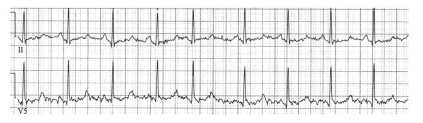

Fig. 8. Hypothermia. These rhythm strips (leads II and V5) are from a patient presenting with mild hypothermia. Sinus rhythm with an underlying tremor artifact is evident.

wave is usually present when the core body temperature falls to less than 32°C (90°F) and is consistently identified when the body temperature falls to less than 25°C (77°F) [31,33]. In one series of 43 patients who were hypothermic, 37 of 43 initial ECGs demonstrated Osborn waves. In this study, Osborn waves were present on all ECGs in patients who had a core body temperature of ≤30.5°C (87.0°F) [34]. The size of the Osborn wave has been shown to correlate directly with the degree of hypothermia. Osborn waves may persist in patients after they have been adequately rewarmed [34]. Osborn waves also have been noted to occur, albeit rarely, in certain normothermic conditions, such as hypercalcemia, massive head injury, and subarachnoid hemorrhage [7].

Atrial fibrillation is another common ECG finding in patients who have hypothermia, occurring in 50%–60% of cases and appearing at a mean body temperature of 29°C (84°F) [33]. In severe hypothermia, marked bradycardia, asystole, and ventricular fibrillation also can occur.

Hyperthyroidism

ECG manifestations of hyperthyroidism frequently are encountered, although no abnormality is pathognomonic for this condition. Sinus tachycardia is the most common cardiac arrhythmia observed in patients who have hyperthyroid conditions and occurs in approximately 40% of cases [1,35]. Atrial fibrillation occurs in 10%–22% of hyperthyroid patients and usually is associated with a rapid ventricular response [35,36]. Although rare in

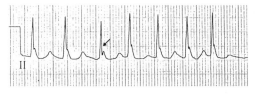

Fig. 9. Osborn waves of hypothermia. This lead II rhythm strip is from a patient with a core body temperature of 32°C (90°F). The rhythm strip demonstrates Osborn waves (*arrow*). These Osborn waves can be huge or subtle; this case is less prominent than some.

patients <40 years of age, atrial fibrillation seems to be more likely to occur in thyrotoxic patients who are older than 60 years of age, male, and have a history of hypertension or rheumatic heart disease [35,36]. The presence of atrial fibrillation, however, should not be uniformly attributed to hyperthyroidism. Its occurrence should prompt an evaluation for the presence of underlying structural heart disease.

Intraventricular conduction disturbances, most commonly a left anterior fascicular block or right bundle branch block, occur in approximately 15% of hyperthyroid patients without underlying heart disease [2]. Nonspecific ST segment/T-wave abnormalities also are noted in 25% of patients [2]. Atrial flutter, supraventricular tachycardia, and ventricular tachycardia are uncommon, however. In patients who have hyperthyroidism, there is also an increased incidence of P wave and PR interval prolongation.

Hypothyroidism

The ECG manifestations of hypothyroidism include sinus bradycardia, low voltage complexes (small P waves or QRS complexes), prolonged PR and QT intervals, and flattened or inverted T waves (Fig. 10) [1,5,6,35]. Pericardial effusions occur in up to 30% of hypothyroid patients and may be responsible for some of the ECG manifestations [5,6]. Atrial, intraventricular, or ventricular conduction disturbances are three times more likely to occur in patients who have myxedema than in the general population [2,6].

Maintenance hemodialysis

When patients who have endstage renal disease (ESRD) receiving hemodialysis (HD) are assessed with a standard 12-lead ECG or 24-hour Holter monitor, a wide range of abnormalities are identified [37,38]. In a study of 221 outpatients receiving maintenance HD, 143 patients (64.7%) had ECG abnormalities, not including sinus tachycardia, sinus bradycardia, or sinus arrhythmia [37]. Common ECG abnormalities that were identified

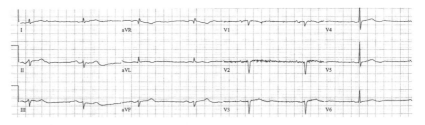

Fig. 10. Myxedematous hypothyroidism. This ECG is from a patient presenting with myxedema coma. The ECG demonstrates sinus bradycardia, low voltage complexes, and T-wave flattening. The thyroid stimulating hormone level was markedly elevated at 40 mIU/mL.

by a standard 12-lead ECG included LVH, PVCs, myocardial ischemia, supraventricular premature contractions (SVPCs), and nonspecific ST segment/ T-wave changes. The ESRD group receiving HD had a much higher rate of ECG abnormalities as compared with non-HD patients who had chronic renal failure and to normal control subjects.

Among the maintenance HD group, males had a higher rate of ECG abnormalities than females (68% vs 53%) and the frequency of abnormalities increased with age. ECG abnormalities were also noted in 70% of patients with hypertension and in 91% of patients with diabetes mellitus. These rates are statistically higher than those HD patients without those diseases. Surprisingly, the prevalence of ECG abnormalities correlated inversely with the duration of time that a patient required HD.

Among the 221 patients receiving maintenance HD, 72 were selected for 24-hour Holter ECG monitoring. Commonly identified abnormalities included SVPCs in 68 patients (94%), PVCs in 62 patients (86%) (of which 9% were multiform), and ST segment/T-wave changes in 43 patients (60%). The physiologic and metabolic changes associated with HD may contribute to the occurrence of ECG abnormalities, because 40% of patients who had PVCs, 27% of patients who had SPVCs, and 26% of patients who had ST segment/T-wave changes occurred during HD and resolved a few hours after the completion of HD.

In another study of 20 patients undergoing maintenance HD as a result of ESRD, ventricular arrhythmias were observed in 18 patients (90%) undergoing 24-hour Holter ECG monitoring [39]. In 15 of these cases, the dysrhythmias were sporadic or isolated, and in three cases they were frequent (multiform, couplets, and salvos). In the study population, ventricular dysrhythmias significantly increased during HD and for 4 hours afterward.

HD also can be associated with an increase in the duration of the QTc interval in patients with ESRD. In a study by Covic and colleagues, QTc intervals were measured 10 minutes before and 10 minutes after HD in 68 nondiabetic ESRD patients without known underlying heart disease [40]. QTc intervals increased post-HD in 47 (69%) patients. In this study population, the major contributor to the increase in the QTc intervals seemed to be changes between the pre-HD and post-HD calcium concentration.

Summary

Alterations in serum calcium and potassium concentration may manifest as detectable changes on the ECG and alert the emergency physician to the presence of an underlying electrolyte disturbance. In addition, various endocrine abnormalities, metabolic disturbances, and environmental emergencies may cause alterations in the ECG.

References

[1] Barsness GW, Feinglos MN. Endocrine systems and the heart. In: Topol EJ, Califf RM, Isner JM, et al, editors. Comprehensive cardiovascular medicine. Baltimore: Lippincott Raven; 1998. p. 952–69.

[2] Kawai C, Nakamura Y. The heart in nutritional disorders. In: Braunwald E, editor. Atlas of heart disease. Vol. II. Cardiomyopathies, myocarditis, and pericardial disease. St. Louis: Mosby; 1995. p. 7.1–7.18.

[3] Fisch C. Electrocardiography and vectorcardiography. In: Braunwald E, editor. Heart disease: A textbook of cardiovascular medicine. 4th edition. Philadelphia: WB Saunders; 1992. p. 116–60.

[4] Marriott HJ. Miscellaneous conditions. In: Marriott HJ, editor. Practical electrocardiography. 8th edition. Philadelphia: Williams & Wilkins; 1988. p. 511–43.

[5] Vela BS, Crawford MH. Endocrinology and the heart. In: Crawford MH, editor. Current diagnosis and treatment in cardiology. New York: Lange Medical Book; 1995. p. 411–27.

[6] Vela BS. Endocrinology and the heart. In: Crawford MH, DiMarco JP, Asplund, et al, editors. Cardiology. St. Louis: Mosby; 2001. p. 4.1–4.13.

[7] Slovis C, Jenkins R. Conditions not primarily affecting the heart. BMJ 2002;324:1320–3.

[8] Chia BL, Thai AC. Electrocardiographic abnormalities in combined hypercalcemia and hypokalemia. Ann Acad Med Singapore 1998;27:567–9.

[9] Surawicz B. Electrolytes and the electrocardiogram. Postgrad Med 1974;55:123–9.

[10] RuDusky BM. ECG abnormalities associated with hypocalcemia. Chest 2001;119:668–9.

[11] Lehman G, Deisenhofer I, Ndrepepa G, et al. ECG changes in a 25-year-old woman with hypocalcemia due to hypoparathyroidism. Chest 2000;118:260–2.

[12] Webster A, Brady W, Morris F. Recognising signs of danger: ECG changes resulting from an abnormal serum potassium concentration. Emerg Med J 2002;19:74–7.

[13] Diercks DB, Shumaik GM, Harrigan RA, et al. Electrocardiographic manifestations: electrolyte abnormalities. J Emerg Med 2004;27:153–60.

[14] Surawicz B, Knilans TK. Electrolytes, temperature, central nervous system diseases and miscellaneous effects. In: Surawicz B, editor. Chou's electrocardiography in clinical practice. 5th edition. Philadelphia: WB Saunders; 2001. p. 516–39.

[15] Mattu A, Brady WJ, Robinson DA. Electrocardiographic manifestations of hyperkalemia. Am J Emerg Med 2000;18:721–9.

[16] Cohen A, Utarnachitt RV. Electrocardiographic changes in a patient with hyperkalemia and diabetic acidosis associated with acute anteroseptal pseudomyocardial infarction and bifascicular block. Angiology 1981;32:361–4.

[17] Lim YH, Anantharaman V. Pseudo myocardial infarct—electrocardiographic pattern in a patient with diabetic ketoacidosis. Singapore Med J 1998;39:504–6.

[18] Pastor JA, Castellanos A, Moleiro F, et al. Patterns of acute inferior wall myocardial infarction caused by hyperkalemia. J Electrocardiol 2001;34:53–8.

[19] Moulik PK, Nethaji C, Khaleeli AA. Misleading electrocardiographic results in patient with hyperkalemia and diabetic ketoacidosis. BMJ 2002;325:1346–7.

[20] Sweterlitsch EM, Murphy GW. Acute electrocardiographic pseudoinfarction pattern in the setting of diabetic ketoacidosis and severe hyperkalemia. Am Heart J 1996;132:1086–9.

[21] Martinez-Vea A, Bardaji A, Garcia C, et al. Severe hyperkalemia with minimal electrocardiographic manifestations. J Electrocardiol 1999;32:45–9.

[22] McGovern B. Hypokalemia and cardiac arrhythmias. Anesthesiology 1985;63:127–9.

[23] Marinella MA, Burdette SD. Hypokalemia induced QT interval prolongation. J Emerg Med 2000;19:375–6.

[24] Pham KNRE. A case of hypokalemia induced QT interval prolongation. J Emerg Med 2001;21:77–8.

[25] Nosworthy A. Images in clinical medicine. Hypokalemia. Engl N. J Med 2003;349:2116.

[26] Jones E. Hypokalemia. N Engl J Med 2003;350:1156.
[27] Clausen TG, Brocks K, Ibsen H. Hypokalemia and ventricular arrhythmias in acute myocardial infarction. Acta Med Scand 1988;224:531–7.
[28] Solomon RJ, Cole AG. Importance of potassium in patients with acute myocardial infarction. Acta Med Scand Suppl 1981;647:87–93.
[29] Nordrehaug JE. Malignant arrhythmia in relation to serum potassium in acute myocardial infarction. Am J Cardiol 1985;56:20D–3.
[30] Helfant RH. Hypokalemia and arrhythmias. Am J Med 1986;25:13–22.
[31] Chou TC. Electrocardiography in clinical practice. 3rd edition. Philadelphia: WB Saunders; 1991. p. 503–8.
[32] Cheng D. The EKG of hypothermia. J Emerg Med 2002;22:87–9.
[33] Mattu A, Brady WJ, Perron AD. Electrocardiographic manifestations of hypothermia. Am J Emerg Med 2002;20:314–26.
[34] Vassallo SU, Delaney KA, Hoffman RS, et al. A prospective evaluation of the electrocardiographic manifestations of hypothermia. Acad Emerg Med 1999;6:1121–6.
[35] Chipkin SR. The thyroid and heart disease. In: Hurst JW, Alpert JS, editors. Diagnostic atlas of the heart. New York: Raven Press; 1994. p. 503–16.
[36] Fadel B, Ellahham S, Ringel MD, et al. Hyperthyroid heart disease. Clin Cardiol 2000;23: 402–8.
[37] Abe S, Yoshizawa M, Nakanishi N, et al. Electrocardiographic abnormalities in patients receiving hemodialysis. Am Heart J 1996;131:1137–40.
[38] Loroincz I, Zilahi Z, Kun C, et al. ECG abnormalities in hemodialysis. Am Heart J 1997;134: 1138–40.
[39] Erem C, Kulan K, Tuncer C, et al. Cardiac arrhythmias in patients on maintenance hemodialysis. Acta Cardiol 1997;52:25–36.
[40] Covic A, Diaconita M, Gusbeth-Tatomir P, et al. Haemodialysis increases QTc interval but not QTc dispersion in ESRD patients without manifest cardiac disease. Nephrol Dial Transplant 2002;17:2170–7.

ELSEVIER
SAUNDERS

EMERGENCY
MEDICINE
CLINICS OF
NORTH AMERICA

Emerg Med Clin N Am 24 (2006) 159–177

ECG Manifestations:
The Poisoned Patient

Christopher P. Holstege, MD*, David L. Eldridge, MD,
Adam K. Rowden, DO

*Division of Medical Toxicology, Department of Emergency Medicine,
University of Virginia, P.O. Box 800774, Charlottesville, VA 22908-0774, USA*

Emergency physicians routinely evaluate and manage poisoned patients. In 2003, more than 2 million human exposure cases were reported to poison centers throughout the United States [1]. Of those cases, 22% were treated in a health care facility with most of those cases evaluated in the emergency department. Cardiovascular drugs were listed as the fifteenth most frequently encountered human exposure (66,401) and the fifth leading cause of poisoning deaths.

Drug-induced changes and abnormalities on the 12-lead electrocardiogram (ECG) are common. There are numerous drugs that can cause ECG changes and lead to cardiac dysrhythmias. The diagnoses and subsequent management of patients manifesting ECG changes following poisonings can challenge even the most experienced physician. Drugs that are advocated in Advanced Coronary Life Support protocols for cardiac dysrhythmias may not apply or may even worsen the condition of overdose patients [2].

Despite that drugs have widely varying indications for therapeutic use, many unrelated drugs share a common cardiac pharmacologic effect if taken in overdose. The purpose of this article is to group together agents that cause similar electrocardiographic effects, review their pharmacologic actions, and discuss the electrocardiographic findings reported in the medical literature. The five main categories reviewed include potassium (K+) efflux blockers, sodium (Na+) channel blockers, sodium-potassium adenosine-triphosphatase (Na+/K+ ATPase) blockers, calcium channel blockers (CCB), and beta-adrenergic blockers (BB). It is important to keep in mind, however, that many medications have actions that involve more than one of these

---

* Corresponding author.
E-mail address: ch2xf@virginia.edu (C.P. Holstege).

actions, and thus may result in a combination or myriad of electrocardio-graphic changes.

Cardiac physiology

To understand the ECG changes associated with various drugs, physicians must have a clear understanding of basic myocardial cell function. The myocardial cell membrane in its resting state is impermeable to Na+ (Fig. 1). The Na+/K+ ATPase actively pumps three sodium ions out of cardiac cells while pumping in two potassium ions to maintain a negative electric potential of approximately 90 mV in the myocyte (phase 4). Depolarization of the cardiac cell membrane is caused by the rapid opening of Na+ channels and subsequent massive Na+ influx (phase 0). This Na+ influx causes the rapid upstroke of the cardiac action potential as it is conducted through the ventricles and is directly responsible for the QRS interval of the ECG. The peak of the action potential is marked by the closure of Na+ channels and the activation of K+ efflux channels (phase 1). Calcium (Ca++) influx then occurs, allowing for a plateau in the action potential (phase 2) and continued myocardial contraction. The cardiac cycle ends with closure of the Ca++ channels and activation of K+ efflux channels, causing the potential to again approach −90 mV (phase 3). It is this potassium efflux from the myocardial cell that is directly responsible for the QT interval on the ECG [3].

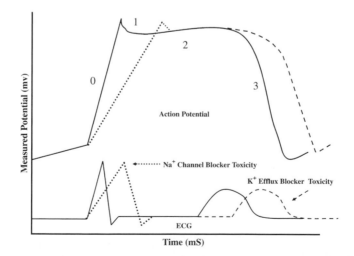

Fig. 1. Cardiac cycle action potential with corresponding electrocardiographic tracing. *Dotted line* indicates the changes associated with Na+ channel blocker toxicity. *Dashed line* indicates the changes associated with K+ efflux blocker toxicity.

Potassium efflux blocker toxicity

Background

Medications in the K+ efflux blocker category are listed in Table 1. These medications all block the outward flow of potassium from intracellular to extracellular spaces. Myocardial repolarization is driven predominantly by this outward movement of potassium ions [3]. Blockade of the outward potassium currents by drugs may prolong the cardiac cycle action potential (Fig. 1) [4]. As a result, the primary electrocardiographic manifestation of potassium efflux blocker toxicity is QT interval prolongation. In fact, studies suggest that approximately 3% of total noncardiac prescriptions are associated with the potential for QT interval prolongation [5].

These medications vary in their propensity to induce QT interval prolongation or associated dysrhythmias at therapeutic and toxic levels. Some of these drugs, such as sotalol, are marketed specifically for their ability to inhibit this delayed rectifier current [6]. Other medications possess this activity as an unwelcome side effect at therapeutic doses. Several medications, such as terfenadine and cisapride, have been removed from the market in various countries because of reports of associated torsades de pointes and sudden death in patients taking these drugs [7,8]. Other medications in this class rarely have been reported to cause QT interval prolongation except when taken in massive overdose.

In addition, many of these drugs have other effects that can result in significant cardiovascular and electrocardiographic changes. For example, antipsychotic agents can cause muscarinic acetylcholine receptor and alpha-adrenergic receptor blockade and cardiac cell potassium, sodium, and calcium channel blockade.

Electrocardiographic manifestations

As noted, the primary electrocardiographic manifestation of K+ efflux blocker toxicity is QT interval prolongation (Fig. 2). When measuring the QT interval, the ECG is best recorded at a paper speed of 50 mm/sec and an amplitude of 0.5 mV/cm (the latter is equal to 20 mm/mV; the usual settings are 25 mm/sec and 10 mm/mV). A tangent line then is drawn to the steepest part of the descending portion of the T wave. The intercept between that line and the isoelectric line is defined as the end of the T wave. The QT interval then is measured from the beginning of the QRS complex to the end of the T wave. Within any ECG tracing, there is lead-to-lead variation of the QT interval. In general, the longest measurable QT interval on an ECG is regarded as determining the overall QT interval for a given tracing [9]. The QT interval is influenced by the patient's heart rate. The RR interval should be measured to allow for rate correction. Several formulas have been developed to correct the QT interval for the effect of heart rate (QTc), with Bazett's formula ($QTc = QT/RR^{1/2}$) being the most commonly

Table 1
K^+ efflux channel blocking drugs

Antihistamines
  Astemizole
  Diphenhydramine
  Loratidine
  Terfenadine
Antipsychotics
  Chlorpromazine
  Droperidol
  Haloperidol
  Mesoridazine
  Pimozide
  Quetiapine
  Risperidone
  Thioridazine
  Ziprasidone
Arsenic trioxide
Bepridil
Chloroquine
Cisapride
Citalopram
Class IA antidysrhythmics
  Disopyramide
  Quinidine
  Procainamide
Class IC antidysrhythmics
  Encainide
  Flecainide
  Moricizine
  Propafenone
Class III antidysrhythmics
  Amiodarone
  Dofetilide
  Ibutilide
  Sotalol
Cyclic antidepressants
  Amitriptyline
  Amoxapine
  Desipramine
  Doxepin
  Imipramine
  Nortriptyline
  Maprotiline
Fluoroquinolones
  Ciprofloxacin
  Gatifloxacin
  Levofloxacin
  Moxifloxacin
  Sparfloxacin
Halofantrine
Hydroxychloroquine
Levomethadyl

Table 1 (*continued*)

Macrolides
Clarithromycin
Erythromycin
Pentamidine
Quinine
Tacrolimus
Venlafaxine

used. QT interval prolongation is considered to occur when the QTc interval is greater than 0.44 seconds in men and 0.46 seconds in women.

The potential risk for QT interval prolongation with this class of medications is not simply related to a drug dose or concentration. Other factors also influence the QT interval, such as the patient's sex and electrolyte concentrations. In addition to QT interval prolongation, there is also the potential emergence of T- or U-wave abnormalities on the ECG with this class of medications [10].

Moreover, delay of repolarization causes the myocardial cell to have less charge difference across its membrane. This change can result in activation of the inward depolarization current (early after-depolarization), which may in turn promote triggered activity. This triggered activity potentially can progress to re-entry and subsequent polymorphic ventricular tachycardia, or torsades de pointes [11]. These dysrhythmias are associated most commonly with QT intervals greater than 0.50 seconds, although the potential for dysrhythmia for a given QT interval varies from drug to drug and patient to patient [3]. In addition, there is not a simple relationship between the degree of drug-induced QT interval prolongation and the potential for

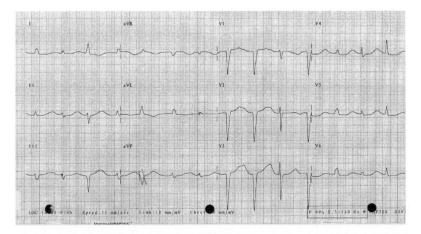

Fig. 2. K+ efflux blocker toxicity. Note the marked QT interval prolongation on this 12-lead ECG; hydroxychloroquine was the offending agent.

the occurrence of torsades de pointes. Drug-induced torsades de pointes can occur even without any substantial prolongation of the QT interval [3].

Similar to other members of this class, antipsychotic agents can cause significant QT interval prolongation and associated dysrhythmias. Additionally, other ECG abnormalities can be seen as a result of other actions of these agents. QRS complex widening can occur as a result of Na+ channel blockade (see later discussion). Sinus tachycardia can occur because of the anticholinergic effect of these medications and from the reflex tachycardia induced by alpha-adrenergic blockade in the peripheral vasculature.

Management

If a patient has drug-induced QT interval prolongation, therapy should focus on immediate withdrawal of the potential cause and correction of any coexisting medical problems, such as electrolyte abnormalities. Patients who have newly diagnosed drug-induced prolongation of their QT interval should be considered candidates for admission to a monitored setting. Intravenous magnesium sulfate is a highly effective and benign intervention to suppress occurrence of dysrhythmias associated with QT interval prolongation, even though it typically does not result in shortening of the QT interval itself [12]. In patients who have intermittent runs of torsades de pointes not responsive to magnesium therapy, electrical overdrive pacing should be considered. In the presence of a non-perfusing rhythm, such as ventricular fibrillation, pulseless ventricular tachycardia, or torsades de pointes, unsynchronized electrical defibrillation should be performed.

Sodium channel blocker toxicity

Background

The ability of drugs to induce cardiac sodium (Na+) channel blockade has been well described in numerous literature reports [13]. This Na+ channel blockade activity has been described as a membrane stabilizing effect, a local anesthetic effect, or a quinidine-like effect. Cardiac voltage-gated sodium channels reside in the cell membrane and open in response to depolarization of the cell (Fig. 1). The Na+ channel blockers bind to the transmembrane Na+ channels and decrease the number available for depolarization. This creates a delay of Na+ entry into the cardiac myocyte during phase 0 of depolarization. As a result, the upslope of depolarization is slowed and the QRS complex widens. Myocardial Na+ channel blocking drugs comprise a diverse group of pharmaceutical agents (Table 2). Specific drugs may affect not only the myocardial Na+ channels, but also other myocardial ion channels, such as the calcium influx and potassium efflux. This may result in ECG changes and rhythm disturbances not related entirely to the drug's Na+ channel blocking activity. For example, sodium

Table 2
Na$^+$ channel blocking drugs

Amantadine
Carbamazepine
Chloroquine
Class IA antidysrhythmics
Disopyramide
Quinidine
Procainamide
Class IC antidysrhythmics
Encainide
Flecainide
Propafenone
Citalopram
Cocaine
Cyclic antidepressants
Amitriptyline
Amoxapine
Desipramine
Doxepin
Imipramine
Nortriptyline
Maprotiline
Diltiazem
Diphenhydramine
Hydroxychloroquine
Loxapine
Orphenadrine
Phenothiazines
Mesoridazine
Thioridazine
Propranolol
Propoxyphene
Quinine
Verapamil

channel blocking medications such as diphenhydramine, propoxyphene, and cocaine also may develop anticholinergic, opioid, and sympathomimetic syndromes, respectively [14–16]. Similarly, cyclic antidepressant toxicity results not only from myocyte sodium channel blockade, but also from their action with respect to alpha-adrenergic blockade, muscarinic anticholinergic effects, and presynaptic neurotransmitter reuptake inhibition.

Electrocardiographic manifestations

As a result of its action in slowing the upslope of depolarization in the cardiac cycle, Na+ channel blockers result in widening of the QRS complex (Fig. 3) [17]. In some cases, the QRS complexes may take the pattern of recognized bundle branch blocks [18,19]. In the most severe cases, the QRS prolongation becomes so profound that it is difficult to distinguish between

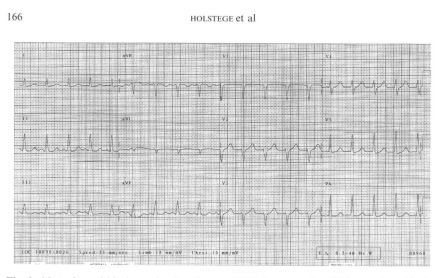

Fig. 3. Na+ channel blocker poisoning. 12-lead ECG demonstrating QRS complex widening and tachycardia as a result of tricyclic antidepressant overdose.

ventricular and supraventricular rhythms [20,21]. Continued prolongation of the QRS complex may result in a sine wave pattern (Fig. 4) and eventual asystole.

Sodium channel blockers also may induce ventricular tachycardia [22]. It has been theorized that the Na+ channel blockers can cause slowed intraventricular conduction, unidirectional block, the development of a reentrant circuit, and a resulting ventricular tachycardia (Fig. 5). These

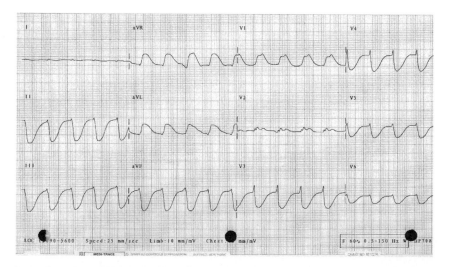

Fig. 4. Na+ channel blocking agent toxicity. 12-lead ECG demonstrating sine wave pattern following overdose; atrial and ventricular activity are difficult to distinguish.

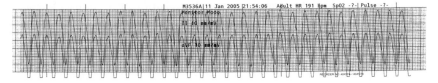

Fig. 5. Wide complex tachydysrhythmia caused by Na+ channel blocker poisoning. ECG rhythm strip revealing a wide complex tachycardia following overdose of diphenhydramine.

rhythms then can degenerate into ventricular fibrillation. Because many of the Na+ channel blocking agents are also anticholinergic or sympathomimetic agents, bradydysrhythmias are rare. The Na+ channel blocking agents, however, can affect cardiac pacemaker cells. Bradycardia may occur because of slowed depolarization of pacemaker cells that depend on entry of sodium ions. In Na+ channel blocker poisoning by anticholinergic and sympathomimetic drugs, the combination of a wide QRS complex and bradycardia is an ominous sign and may indicate that the Na+ channel blockade is so profound that tachycardia does not occur, despite clinical muscarinic antagonism or adrenergic agonism [13].

In this class of agents, cyclic antidepressants produce several ECG changes related to Na+ channel blockade and their other actions on cardiovascular function (see Fig. 3). Sinus tachycardia occurs frequently from the anticholinergic effects of cyclic antidepressant toxicity. QRS complex widening occurs as a result of Na+ blockade, and this delayed conduction may be seen more commonly involving the right side of the heart, manifesting as a right bundle branch block [23]. In addition, QT interval prolongation can occur with these agents. Finally, rightward axis deviation of the terminal 40 msec (0.04 seconds) of the frontal plane QRS axis has been associated with tricyclic antidepressant poisoning [24,25]. The occurrence of this finding in other Na+ channel blocking agents is unknown.

Cocaine is a unique sympathomimetic agent in its ability to cause cardiac Na+ channel blockade. Together with QRS complex widening, increased catecholamine activity seen with cocaine toxicity can result in several rhythm disturbances, including sinus tachycardia, premature ventricular contractions, wide complex dysrhythmias, ventricular tachycardia, and ventricular fibrillation. In addition, morphologic changes in the ST segment and T waves consistent with ischemia can be seen in the setting of sympathomimetic and cocaine toxicity.

Management

The management of Na+ channel blocking agents consists of administration of sodium or creation of an alkalosis [26–30]. Infusion of sodium bicarbonate by intermittent bolus or by continuous infusion has been advocated. Hypertonic sodium infusion and hyperventilation also have been advocated

[31–34]. Reasonable, literature-supported indications for sodium bicarbonate infusion include a QRS duration of >0.10 seconds, persistent hypotension despite adequate hydration, and ventricular dysrhythmias. Lidocaine has been suggested in the treatment of ventricular dysrhythmias, though clear evidence is lacking. Class IA and IC antidysrhythmics should be avoided because of their ability to block cardiac sodium channels.

Sodium–potassium ATPase blocker toxicity

Background

Cardiac glycosides are agents that inhibit the sodium–potassium adenosine triphosphatase (Na+/K+ ATPase) pump. Digoxin and other digitalis derivatives are the cardiac glycosides encountered most widely, but numerous other similar acting agents also exist (Box 1). Digoxin historically has been administered to treat supraventricular tachydysrhythmias and congestive heart failure, but its use has been decreasing as newer agents have been developed. Nonprescription medication cardiac glycosides also have been associated with human toxicity, such as after ingestion of specific plants and contaminated herbal products [35–40].

The cardiac glycosides inhibit active transport of Na+ and K+ across cell membranes by inhibiting the Na+/K+ ATPase. This results in an increase in extracellular K+ and intracellular Na+. An increased intracellular Na+ reduces the transmembrane Na+ gradient and subsequent increased activity of the Na+–Ca^{2+} exchanger. This activity, in turn, increases the intracellular calcium concentration, which then augments myofibril activity in cardiac myocytes and results in a positive inotropic effect. The cardiac glycosides also increase vagal tone that may lead to a direct atrioventricular (AV) nodal depression. Therapeutically, digitalis derivatives are used to increase myocardial contractility or slow AV conduction. These actions, however, can result in significant cardiac disturbances and ECG abnormalities in the setting of toxicity.

Box 1. Na+/K+ ATPase blocking agents and substances

Bufadienolides
Digoxin
Digitoxin
Foxglove
Lily of the valley
Oleander
Red squill

Electrocardiographic manifestations

Digitalis derivatives at therapeutic doses have been associated with several electrocardiographic changes. These findings include the so-called "digitalis effect" manifesting with abnormal inverted or flattened T waves coupled with ST segment depression, frequently described as a sagging or scooped ST segment/T wave complex. These findings are most pronounced in leads with tall R waves. In addition, other findings include QT interval shortening as a result of decreased ventricular repolarization time, PR interval lengthening as a result of increased vagal activity, and increased U-wave amplitude. It is important to remember that these electrocardiographic manifestations are seen with therapeutic digoxin levels and do not correlate with toxicity.

Electrocardiographic abnormalities with cardiac glycoside toxicity are the result of the propensity for increased automaticity (from increased intracellular calcium) accompanied by slowed conduction through the AV node. As a result, cardiac glycoside toxicity may result in a wide array of dysrhythmias [41,42]. Excitant activity (atrial, junctional, and ventricular premature beats, tachydysrhythmias, and triggered dysrhythmias), suppressant activity (sinus bradycardia, bundle branch blocks, first-, second-, and third-degree AV blocks), and any combination of excitant and suppressant activity (atrial tachycardia with AV block, second-degree AV block with junctional premature beats) have all been reported (Fig. 6) [43–45].

The most common dysrhythmia associated with toxicity induced by these agents is frequent premature ventricular beats [42]. Paroxysmal atrial tachycardia with variable block or accelerated junctional rhythm is highly suggestive of digitalis toxicity. Marked slowing of the ventricular response in a patient who has atrial fibrillation who is on digoxin should suggest the possibility of toxicity (Fig. 6). Bidirectional ventricular tachycardia is stated to be specific for digitalis toxicity, but rarely is seen [46].

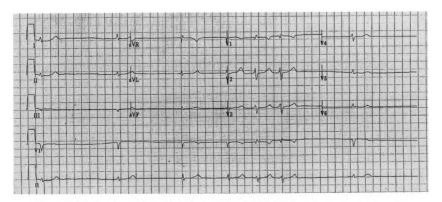

Fig. 6. Na+/K+ ATPase blocker toxicity. 12-lead ECG demonstrating an irregular bradydysrhythmia as a result of conduction block from chronic digoxin toxicity.

The ECG may demonstrate findings associated not only with cardiac glycoside toxicity but also with hyperkalemia. Acute toxicity most closely correlates with hyperkalemia as the Na+/K+ ATPase is inhibited and extracellular K+ increases. In chronic toxicity, hyperkalemia may not be seen because of the slower increase in K+, allowing for renal compensation.

Management

In cardiac glycoside toxicity, digoxin-specific antibody (Fab) fragments are the first-line therapy in patients who have symptomatic cardiac dysrhythmias [41,47]. Because cardiac glycoside-enhanced vagal activity may be reversed by atropine sulfate, this agent has been used successfully in patients exhibiting AV block on ECG [48]. Cardiac pacing has been advocated for bradydysrhythmias unresponsive to atropine, but care should be exercised as the pacing wire itself may induce ventricular fibrillation [49]. The classic antidysrhythmic of choice for ventricular dysrhythmias is phenytoin, because it increases the ventricular fibrillation threshold in the myocardium and enhances conduction through the AV node [41]. Quinidine and procainamide are contraindicated because they depress AV nodal conduction and may worsen cardiac toxicity [50].

Calcium channel blocker toxicity

Background

There are currently nine cardiac calcium channel blockers (CCBs) that have been approved for clinical use in the United States. These nine are subclassified within four classes of compounds (Box 2). Over the past decade,

---

Box 2. Ca^{++} channel blocking drugs

Dihydropyridines
   Nicardipine
   Nifedipine
   Isradipine
   Amlodipine
   Felodipine
   Nimodipine
Phenylalkylamine
   Verapamil
Benzothiazepine
   Diltiazem
Diarylaminopropylamine ether
   Bepridil

the number of exposures to these agents has increased dramatically as they have become available on the market. In 2001, CCBs accounted for 40% of all the deaths caused by cardiovascular drugs reported to the AAPCC [51].

All cardiac CCBs inhibit the voltage sensitive L-type calcium channel within the cell membrane [52]. This channel resides in heart and smooth muscle cell membranes. The inhibition of this channel prevents movement of calcium from extracellular sites through the cell membrane to intracellular sites. Decreased intracellular calcium within the myocardial cells results in slowing of conduction, decreased contractility, and decreased cardiac output.

Blockade of calcium influx within the vascular smooth muscle cells results in vasodilation. Decreased cardiac output coupled with vasodilation can result in profound hypotension. The dihydropyridine class of drugs tends to have a higher affinity for the peripheral vascular smooth muscle cells, less effect on the cardiac calcium channels, and is associated more often with hypotension with a resulting reflex tachycardia. Verapamil and diltiazem, on the other hand, have strong affinity for cardiac and vascular calcium channels and subsequently the combination of hypotension with bradycardia may be seen. In animal models and human case series, CCBs also have been associated with cardiac sodium channel blockade [53,54].

Electrocardiographic manifestations

The inhibition of calcium influx within the conduction system results in slowing of cardiac conduction. CCB toxicity initially causes a sinus bradycardia that may or may not be symptomatic. Depending on the agent ingested, reflex tachycardia may not be seen. As levels of CCB increase, the patient may develop various degrees of AV block (first-, second-, and third-degree) and junctional and ventricular bradydysrhythmias on ECG (Fig. 7). A widening of the QRS complex may be encountered. This may be caused by ventricular escape rhythms or by CCB-induced sodium channel blockade causing a delay of phase 0 of depolarization. This delay and subsequent QRS complex widening also increases the potential for dysrhythmias (see the previous section on Sodium channel blocker toxicity)

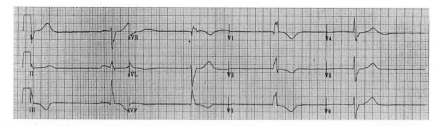

Fig. 7. CCB toxicity. 12-lead ECG demonstrating a marked bradydysrhythmia with a heart rate in the thirties.

[53,54]. In the final stages, asystole may occur. Sudden shifts from brady-dysrhythmias to cardiac arrest have been reported [53]. In addition, ECG changes associated with cardiac ischemia may occur as a result of the hypotension and changes in cardiovascular status, particularly in patients who have pre-existing cardiac disease.

Management

A symptomatic acute CCB overdose can be one of the most challenging poisonings encountered by a physician. CCB poisonings are prone to developing severe bradydysrhythmias and hypotension and other complications, including pulmonary edema and heart failure [55]. Specific pharmacologic therapy includes the use of atropine, calcium, glucagon, insulin, sodium bicarbonate, or various catecholamines [56,57].

Beta-adrenergic blocker toxicity

Background

BBs are used increasingly because of their efficacy in the treatment of hypertension, ischemic heart disease, and dysrhythmias. BBs competitively inhibit various β-adrenergic receptors. Inhibition of β_1-receptors results in a decrease in the force and rate of myocardial contraction, a decrease in AV nodal conduction velocity, and a decrease in renin secretion. Inhibition of β_2-receptors results in a decrease in glycogenolysis, decrease in gluconeogenesis, and decrease in relaxation of smooth muscles in blood vessels, bronchi, and the gastrointestinal tract. There are currently numerous BBs available (Box 3). These agents share in common the mechanism of

---

Box 3. Beta-adrenergic blocking drugs

Acebutolol
Atenolol
Betaxolol
Bisoprolol
Carvedilol
Esmolol
Labetalol
Metoprolol
Nadolol
Pindolol
Propranolol
Sotalol
Timolol

competitive β-adrenergic receptor antagonism. Some of these agents have equal affinity for β_1 and β_2 receptors (eg, propranolol), whereas others are selective and have greater β_1 than β_2 receptor blocking activity (eg, metoprolol). Some agents also block other receptors, such as α-adrenergic receptors (eg, labetalol), cardiac sodium channels (eg, propranolol, acebutolol), and cardiac potassium efflux channels (eg, sotalol) [58,59].

Electrocardiographic manifestations

In acute overdose, the most pronounced effects of BBs are on the cardiovascular system [60]. Bradycardia (from decreased sinoatrial node function), varying degrees of AV block, and hypotension are generally the hallmarks of significant beta-blocker toxicity. One prospective study attempted to characterize electrocardiographic findings in symptomatic BB overdose [61]. Only 3 of 13 symptomatic patients had bradycardia on their initial ECG (performed while they were classified as symptomatic). First-degree AV block was common, however. In fact, 10 of 12 symptomatic patients with a measurable PR interval (the thirteenth patient had atrial fibrillation) demonstrated a first-degree AV block and had a mean PR interval of 0.22 seconds. This finding was the most common abnormality to be found on electrocardiograms in this symptomatic patient group.

Besides bradycardia and AV block, there are other specific findings that can be seen with individual members within this group of medications. Propranolol is unique because of its Na+ channel blocking activity in overdose that can result in a prolonged QRS interval (>0.10 seconds) [58,61–63]. Propranolol overdose has been associated with a higher mortality rate compared with other BBs [66]. These same investigators also found that a QRS interval >0.10 seconds in these patients was predictive of propranolol-induced seizures. Sotalol is a unique BB in that it possesses the ability to block delayed rectifier potassium channels in a dose-dependent fashion [64]. Acebutolol preferentially blocks β_1 receptors and possesses partial agonist activity and membrane stabilizing activity similar to propranolol. QRS interval widening on ECG and ventricular tachycardia have been reported in several cases [59,65,66].

Management

Specific pharmacologic therapy for BB toxicity may include atropine, glucagon, calcium, insulin, or various catecholamines [67]. Atropine may be considered in an attempt to reverse bradycardia, but has been shown to have poor effect and no impact on blood pressure. Glucagon infusion, which increases intracellular cAMP, should be considered in symptomatic BB toxic patients [60]. Calcium has been shown to have efficacy at reversing the hypotensive effects of BB toxicity in animal models and human case reports [60,68]. Insulin infusions have been advocated for BB toxicity based on an animal model [69]. Catecholamine infusions may be considered after the therapies discussed previously fail to give adequate response. Pacemaker insertion, balloon pump, and bypass all may be considered in cases not responding to pharmacologic therapy.

Summary

Toxicologic, medication- and drug-induced changes and abnormalities on the 12-lead electrocardiogram (ECG) are common. A wide variety of electrocardiographic changes can be seen with cardiac and noncardiac agents and may occur at therapeutic or toxic drug levels. In many instances, however, a common mechanism affecting the cardiac cycle action potential underlies most of these electrocardiographic findings. Knowledge and understanding of these mechanisms and their related affect on the 12-lead ECG can assist the physician in determining those ECG abnormalities associated with specific toxidromes.

References

[1] Watson WA, Litovitz TL, Klein-Schwartz W, et al. 2003 annual report of the American Association of Poison Control Centers Toxic Exposure Surveillance System. Am J Emerg Med 2004;22(5):335–404.
[2] Albertson TE, Dawson A, de Latorre F, et al. TOX-ACLS: toxicologic-oriented advanced cardiac life support. Ann Emerg Med 2001;37(4 Suppl):S78–90.
[3] Yap YG, Camm AJ. Drug induced QT prolongation and torsades de pointes. Heart 2003; 89(11):1363–72.
[4] Anderson ME, Al-Khatib SM, Roden DM, et al. Cardiac repolarization: current knowledge, critical gaps, and new approaches to drug development and patient management. Am Heart J 2002;144(5):769–81.
[5] De Ponti F, Poluzzi E, Montanaro N, et al. QTc and psychotropic drugs. Lancet 2000; 356(9223):75–6.
[6] Munro P, Graham C. Torsades de pointes. Emerg Med J 2002;19(5):485–6.
[7] Kyrmizakis DE, Chimona TS, Kanoupakis EM, et al. QT prolongation and torsades de pointes associated with concurrent use of cisapride and erythromycin. Am J Otolaryngol 2002;23(5):303–7.
[8] Horowitz BZ, Bizovi K, Moreno R. Droperidol—behind the black box warning. Acad Emerg Med 2002;9(6):615–8.
[9] Chan T, Brady W, Harrigan R, et al, eds. ECG in emergency medicine and acute care. Philadelphia: Elsevier-Mosby; 2005.
[10] Sides GD. QT interval prolongation as a biomarker for torsades de pointes and sudden death in drug development. Dis Markers 2002;18(2):57–62.
[11] Nelson LS. Toxicologic myocardial sensitization. J Toxicol Clin Toxicol 2002;40(7):867–79.
[12] Kaye P, O'Sullivan I. The role of magnesium in the emergency department. Emerg Med J 2002;19(4):288–91.
[13] Kolecki PF, Curry SC. Poisoning by sodium channel blocking agents. Crit Care Clin 1997; 13(4):829–48.
[14] Zareba W, Moss AJ, Rosero SZ, et al. Electrocardiographic findings in patients with diphenhydramine overdose. Am J Cardiol 1997;80(9):1168–73.

[15] Stork CM, Redd JT, Fine K, et al. Propoxyphene-induced wide QRS complex dysrhythmia responsive to sodium bicarbonate—a case report. J Toxicol Clin Toxicol 1995;33(2): 179–83.

[16] Kerns W II, Garvey L, Owens J. Cocaine-induced wide complex dysrhythmia. J Emerg Med 1997;15(3):321–9.

[17] Harrigan RA, Brady WJ. ECG abnormalities in tricyclic antidepressant ingestion. Am J Emerg Med 1999;17(4):387–93.

[18] Heaney RM. Left bundle branch block associated with propoxyphene hydrochloride poisoning. Ann Emerg Med 1983;12(12):780–2.

[19] Fernandez-Quero L, Riesgo MJ, Agusti S, et al. Left anterior hemiblock, complete right bundle branch block and sinus tachycardia in maprotiline poisoning. Intensive Care Med 1985; 11(4):220–2.

[20] Brady WJ, Skiles J. Wide QRS complex tachycardia: ECG differential diagnosis. Am J Emerg Med 1999;17(4):376–81.

[21] Clark RF, Vance MV. Massive diphenhydramine poisoning resulting in a wide-complex tachycardia: successful treatment with sodium bicarbonate. Ann Emerg Med 1992;21(3): 318–21.

[22] Joshi AK, Sljapic T, Borghei H, et al. Case of polymorphic ventricular tachycardia in diphenhydramine poisoning. J Cardiovasc Electrophysiol 2004;15(5):591–3.

[23] Liebelt EL, Francis PD, Woolf AD. ECG lead in aVR versus QRS interval in predicting seizures and arrhythmias in acute tricyclic antidepressant toxicity. Ann Emerg Med 1995;26: 195–201.

[24] Wolfe TR, Caravati EM, Rollins DE. Terminal 40-ms frontal plane QRS axis as a marker for tricyclic antidepressant overdose. Ann Emerg Med 1989;18(4):348–51.

[25] Berkovitch M, Matsui D, Fogelman R, et al. Assessment of the terminal 40-millisecond QRS vector in children with a history of tricyclic antidepressant ingestion. Pediatr Emerg Care 1995;11(2):75–7.

[26] Kerr GW, McGuffie AC, Wilkie S. Tricyclic antidepressant overdose: a review. Emerg Med J 2001;18(4):236–41.

[27] Wilson LD, Shelat C. Electrophysiologic and hemodynamic effects of sodium bicarbonate in a canine model of severe cocaine intoxication. J Toxicol Clin Toxicol 2003;41(6):777–88.

[28] Sharma AN, Hexdall AH, Chang EK, et al. Diphenhydramine-induced wide complex dysrhythmia responds to treatment with sodium bicarbonate. Am J Emerg Med 2003;21(3): 212–5.

[29] Bou-Abboud E, Nattel S. Relative role of alkalosis and sodium ions in reversal of class I antiarrhythmic drug-induced sodium channel blockade by sodium bicarbonate. Circulation 1996;94(8):1954–61.

[30] Beckman KJ, Parker RB, Hariman RJ, et al. Hemodynamic and electrophysiological actions of cocaine. Effects of sodium bicarbonate as an antidote in dogs. Circulation 1991;83(5): 1799–807.

[31] McKinney PE, Rasmussen R. Reversal of severe tricyclic antidepressant-induced cardiotoxicity with intravenous hypertonic saline solution. Ann Emerg Med 2003;42(1):20–4.

[32] McCabe JL, Cobaugh DJ, Menegazzi JJ, et al. Experimental tricyclic antidepressant toxicity: a randomized, controlled comparison of hypertonic saline solution, sodium bicarbonate, and hyperventilation. Ann Emerg Med 1998;32(3 Pt 1):329–33.

[33] Hoffman JR, Votey SR, Bayer M, et al. Effect of hypertonic sodium bicarbonate in the treatment of moderate-to-severe cyclic antidepressant overdose. Am J Emerg Med 1993;11(4): 336–41.

[34] Hoegholm A, Clementsen P. Hypertonic sodium chloride in severe antidepressant overdosage. J Toxicol Clin Toxicol 1991;29(2):297–8.

[35] Eddleston M, Ariaratnam CA, Sjostrom L, et al. Acute yellow oleander (*Thevetia peruviana*) poisoning: cardiac arrhythmias, electrolyte disturbances, and serum cardiac glycoside concentrations on presentation to hospital. Heart 2000;83(3):301–6.

[36] Deaths associated with a purported aphrodisiac—New York City, February 1993–May 1995. MMWR Morb Mortal Wkly Rep 1995;44(46):853–5, 861.

[37] Gowda RM, Cohen RA, Khan IA. Toad venom poisoning: resemblance to digoxin toxicity and therapeutic implications. Heart 2003;89(4):e14.

[38] Gupta A, Joshi P, Jortani SA, et al. A case of nondigitalis cardiac glycoside toxicity. Ther Drug Monit 1997;19(6):711–4.

[39] Maringhini G, Notaro L, Barberi O, et al. Cardiovascular glycoside-like intoxication following ingestion of *Thevetia nereifolia/peruviana* seeds: a case report. Ital Heart J 2002;3(2): 137–40.

[40] Scheinost ME. Digoxin toxicity in a 26-year-old woman taking an herbal dietary supplement. J Am Osteopath Assoc 2001;101(8):444–6.

[41] Irwin J. Intensive care medicine. In: Kirk M, Judge B, editors. Digitalis poisoning. 5th edition. Baltimore: Lippincott Williams & Wilkins; 2003.

[42] Ma G, Brady WJ, Pollack M, et al. Electrocardiographic manifestations: digitalis toxicity. J Emerg Med 2001;20(2):145–52.

[43] Chen JY, Liu PY, Chen JH, et al. Safety of transvenous temporary cardiac pacing in patients with accidental digoxin overdose and symptomatic bradycardia. Cardiology 2004;102(3): 152–5.

[44] Harrigan RA, Perron AD, Brady WJ. Atrioventricular dissociation. Am J Emerg Med 2001; 19(3):218–22.

[45] Behringer W, Sterz F, Domanovits H, et al. Percutaneous cardiopulmonary bypass for therapy resistant cardiac arrest from digoxin overdose. Resuscitation 1998;37(1):47–50.

[46] Lien WC, Huang CH, Chen WJ. Bidirectional ventricular tachycardia resulting from digoxin and amiodarone treatment of rapid atrial fibrillation. Am J Emerg Med 2004;22(3):235–6.

[47] Woolf AD, Wenger T, Smith TW, et al. The use of digoxin-specific Fab fragments for severe digitalis intoxication in children. N Engl J Med 1992;326(26):1739–44.

[48] Kaplanski J, Weinhouse E, Martin O. Modification of digoxin induced arrhythmogenicity in adult rats following atropine administration. Res Commun Chem Pathol Pharmacol 1983; 39(1):173–6.

[49] Cummins RO, Haulman J, Quan L, et al. Near-fatal yew berry intoxication treated with external cardiac pacing and digoxin-specific FAB antibody fragments. Ann Emerg Med 1990; 19(1):38–43.

[50] Mordel A, Halkin H, Zulty L, et al. Quinidine enhances digitalis toxicity at therapeutic serum digoxin levels. Clin Pharmacol Ther 1993;53(4):457–62.

[51] Litovitz TL, Klein-Schwartz W, Rodgers GC Jr, et al. 2001 annual report of the American Association of Poison Control Centers Toxic Exposure Surveillance System. Am J Emerg Med 2002;20(5):391–452.

[52] Goldfrank L Goldfrank's toxicologic emergencies. In: DeRoos F, editor. Calcium channel blockers. 7th edition. New York: McGraw-Hill; 2002.

[53] Holstege C, Kirk M, Furbee R. Wide complex dysrhythmia in calcium channel blocker overdose responsive to sodium bicarbonate therapy [abstract]. J Toxicol Clin Toxicol 1998;36(5): 509.

[54] Tanen DA, Ruha AM, Curry SC, et al. Hypertonic sodium bicarbonate is effective in the acute management of verapamil toxicity in a swine model. Ann Emerg Med 2000;36(6): 547–53.

[55] Sami-Karti S, Ulusoy H, Yandi M, et al. Non-cardiogenic pulmonary oedema in the course of verapamil intoxication. Emerg Med J 2002;19(5):458–9.

[56] Kline JA, Tomaszewski CA, Schroeder JD, et al. Insulin is a superior antidote for cardiovascular toxicity induced by verapamil in the anesthetized canine. J Pharmacol Exp Ther 1993; 267(2):744–50.

[57] Kline JA, Leonova E, Raymond RM. Beneficial myocardial metabolic effects of insulin during verapamil toxicity in the anesthetized canine. Crit Care Med 1995;23(7):1251–63.

[58] Love JN, Howell JM, Newsome JT, et al. The effect of sodium bicarbonate on propranolol-induced cardiovascular toxicity in a canine model. J Toxicol Clin Toxicol 2000;38(4):421–8.

[59] Donovan KD, Gerace RV, Dreyer JF. Acebutolol-induced ventricular tachycardia reversed with sodium bicarbonate. J Toxicol Clin Toxicol 1999;37(4):481–4.

[60] Snook CP, Sigvaldason K, Kristinsson J. Severe atenolol and diltiazem overdose. J Toxicol Clin Toxicol 2000;38(6):661–5.

[61] Love JN, Enlow B, Howell JM, et al. Electrocardiographic changes associated with beta-blocker toxicity. Ann Emerg Med 2002;40(6):603–10.

[62] Reith DM, Dawson AH, Epid D, et al. Relative toxicity of beta blockers in overdose. J Toxicol Clin Toxicol 1996;34(3):273–8.

[63] Buiumsohn A, Eisenberg ES, Jacob H, et al. Seizures and intraventricular conduction defect in propranolol poisoning. A report of two cases. Ann Intern Med 1979;91(6):860–2.

[64] Neuvonen PJ, Elonen E, Tarssanen L. Sotalol intoxication, two patients with concentration-effect relationships. Acta Pharmacol Toxicol (Copenh) 1979;45(1):52–7.

[65] Sangster B, de Wildt D, van Dijk A, et al. A case of acebutolol intoxication. J Toxicol Clin Toxicol 1983;20(1):69–77.

[66] Long RR, Sargent JC, Hammer K. Paralytic shellfish poisoning: a case report and serial electrophysiologic observations. Neurology 1990;40(8):1310–2.

[67] Goldfrank L. Goldfrank's toxicologic emergencies. In: Brubacher J, editor. Beta-adrenergic blockers. 7th edition. New York: McGraw-Hill; 2002.

[68] Love JN, Hanfling D, Howell JM. Hemodynamic effects of calcium chloride in a canine model of acute propranolol intoxication. Ann Emerg Med 1996;28(1):1–6.

[69] Kearns W, Schroeder D, Williams C, et al. Insulin improves survival in a canine model of acute beta-blocker toxicity. Ann Emerg Med 1997;29(6):748–57.

ELSEVIER
SAUNDERS

Emerg Med Clin N Am 24 (2006) 179–194

EMERGENCY
MEDICINE
CLINICS OF
NORTH AMERICA

Electronic Pacemakers

Theodore C. Chan, MD*, Taylor Y. Cardall, MD

*Clinical Medicine and Department of Emergency Medicine, University of California,
200 West Arbor Drive #8676, San Diego, CA, USA*
Scottsdale Healthcare, 7400 East Osborn, Scottsdale, AZ, USA

The number of patients who have cardiac pacemakers has increased markedly over the past few decades since the technology was first introduced in the 1950s to prevent Stokes-Adams attacks. The American College of Cardiology and the American Heart Association's Guidelines for Permanent Cardiac Pacemaker Implantation now lists atrioventricular (AV) node dysfunction, sinus node dysfunction, hypersensitive carotid sinus syndrome, and neurally-mediated syncope (vasovagal syncope), the prevention of tachycardia with long QT syndrome, and hypertrophic cardiomyopathy as indications for permanent cardiac pacing [1]. Recent literature expands the list to include select patients who have congestive heart failure and for the prevention of atrial fibrillation. Advances in technology, expanding indications, and the aging of the population ensure that clinicians will encounter patients with cardiac pacemakers on a regular basis. This article summarizes the electrocardiographic manifestations of the normally functioning permanent cardiac pacemaker, as well as abnormalities associated with pacemaker malfunction.

Pacing modes

As pacemakers have evolved and assumed more functions and capabilities, a five position code has been developed by the North American Society of Pacing and Electrophysiology (NASPE) and the British Pacing and Electrophysiology Group (BPEG) to describe pacemaker function [2] (Table 1).

Position I indicates the chambers being paced, atrium (A), ventricle (V), both (D, dual), or none (O). Position II gives the location where the pacemaker senses native cardiac electrical activity (A, V, D, or O). Position III

---

* Corresponding author.
E-mail address: tcchan@ucsd.edu (T.C. Chan).

0733-8627/06/$ - see front matter © 2005 Elsevier Inc. All rights reserved.
doi:10.1016/j.emc.2005.08.011   *emed.theclinics.com*

Table 1
The NASPE/BPEG Generic (NBG) pacemaker code

Position	I	II	III	IV	V
	Chamber(s) paced	Chamber(s) sensed	Response to sensing	Programmability, rate modulation	Antitachy-dysrhythmia functions
	O = none	O = none	O = none	O = none	O = none
	A = atrium	A = atrium	T = triggered	P = simple programmable	P = pacing (antidysrhythmia)
	V = ventricle	V = ventricle	I = inhibited	M = multiprogrammable	S = shock
	D = dual (atrium and ventricle)	D = dual (atrium and ventricle)	D = dual (inhibited and triggered)	C = communicating	D = dual (pacing and shock)
				R = rate modulation	

indicates the pacemaker's response to sensing—triggering (T), inhibition (I), both (D), or none (O). Older versions of the code only designated these three positions, and pacemakers still are commonly referred to in terms of these three codes. Position IV indicates two things: the programmability of the pacemaker and the capability to adaptively control rate (R). The code in this position is hierarchical. The C, which designates the ability to communicate with external equipment (ie, telemetry), thus is assumed to have multiprogrammable capability (M). Similarly, a pacemaker able to modulate rate of pacing (R) is assumed to be able to communicate (C) and be multiprogrammable (M). Position V identifies the presence of antitachydysrhythmia functions, including the antitachydysrhythmia pacing (P) or shocking (S). The code does not designate how these functions are activated or if they are activated automatically or manually by an external command.

For example, a VOOOO pacemaker is one capable of asynchronous ventricular pacing, with no sensing functions, no adaptive rate control functions, and no antitachydysrhythmia capability. A VVIPP pacemaker paces the ventricle, is inhibited in response to sensed ventricular activity, has simple programmability, and has antitachydysrhythmia-pacing capability. Similarly, a VVIMD pacemaker is a multiprogrammable VVI pacemaker with the ability to pace and shock in the setting of a tachydysrhythmia. A DDDCO pacemaker is a DDD pacemaker with telemetry capability but no antitachydysrhythmia function. From a practical standpoint, most pacemakers encountered in the emergency department or clinic setting are AAIR, VVIR, DDD, DDDR, or back-up pacing modes for cardioverter-defibrillator devices.

Electrocardiographic findings in a normally functioning pacemaker

When a pacemaker is active and pacing, small spikes that signify the electrical signal emanating from the pacemaker leads are usually evident on the electrocardiogram (ECG). These low-amplitude pacemaker artifacts may not be visible in all leads. Pacing artifacts are much smaller with bipolar electrode systems than with unipolar leads, and consequently may be difficult to visualize.

Typically, pacing leads used to pace the atrium are implanted in the appendage of the right atrium and leads to pace the ventricles toward the apex of the right ventricle. Atrial pacing appears as a small pacemaker spike just before the P wave. The P wave is usually of a normal morphology. In contrast, the ventricular paced rhythm (VPR) is abnormal (Fig. 1). Because the ventricular pacing lead is placed in the right ventricle, the ventricles contract from right to left, rather than by the regular conduction system. The overall QRS morphology thus is similar to that of a left bundle branch block (LBBB), with prolongation of the QRS interval. In leads V1–V6, the altered ventricular conduction is manifested by wide, mainly negative QS or rS

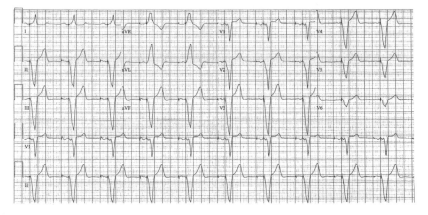

Fig. 1. DDD pacemaker with atrial and ventricular pacing. Low amplitude atrial and ventricular pacing spikes are best seen in lead V1 and II rhythm strips. The tracing demonstrates the widened QRS complexes typical in ventricular-paced rhythm with a left bundle branch block pattern, left axis deviation and ST segment/T-wave discordance with the QRS complex.

complexes with poor R-wave progression. QS complexes are seen commonly in leads II, III, and aVF, whereas a large R-wave typically is seen in leads I and aVL. Leads V5 and V6 sometimes have deep S-waves because the depolarization may be traveling away from the plane of those leads. Usually the ventricular lead is placed near the apex, causing the ventricles to contract from apex to base, yielding leftward deviation of the QRS axis on the ECG. If the lead is implanted toward the right ventricular outflow tract, depolarization forces travel from base to apex, resulting in a right axis deviation. Occasionally patients have epicardial rather than intracardiac pacemaker leads. If the ventricular epicardial lead is placed over the left ventricle, the ventricular paced pattern is that of a right bundle branch block.

ST segments and T waves typically should be discordant with the QRS complex, in contrast to the usual ECG pattern—meaning the major vector of the QRS complex is in a direction opposite that of the ST segment/T-wave complex. This is known as the rule of appropriate discordance or QRS complex/T-wave axis discordance for ventricular pacing. This becomes relevant when interpreting the electrocardiogram with VPR in the context of possible cardiac ischemia [3,4].

AAI pacing

An AAI pacemaker is one that paces the atrium, senses the atrium, and inhibits the pacing activity if it senses spontaneous atrial activity (Fig. 2). This mode of pacing prevents the atrial rate from decreasing below a preset level and is useful for patients who have sinus node dysfunction and intact AV node conduction. The timing cycle of the pacemaker begins when it paces the atrium or senses an atrial event. Following initiation of the timing

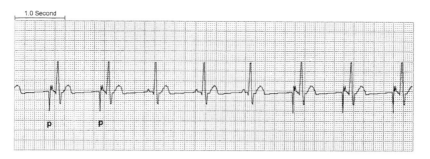

Fig. 2. AAI pacing. The first two P waves are paced (*p*), whereas the following three P waves are native and sensed, so atrial pacing is inhibited. The next three P waves are again paced. *From* Chan TC, et al., eds. ECG in Emergency Medicine and Acute Care. Philadelphia: Mosby, 2004; with permission.

cycle, there is a refractory period in which the pacemaker is insensitive to stimuli. This prevents the pacemaker from sensing the proximate QRS complex and misinterpreting it as an atrial event. Once the preprogrammed refractory period is over, the pacemaker resets to its baseline status and the pacemaker remains silent for the duration of the programmed pacing interval. If, at the end of the interval no atrial activity is sensed, it generates a stimulus and the cycle begins anew. If, following the refractory period, it senses atrial activity, it inhibits itself from stimulating the atrium, and the sensed atrial activity initiates a new timing cycle.

VVI pacing

VVI pacing is useful in patients who have chronically ineffective atria, such as chronic atrial fibrillation or atrial flutter (Fig. 3). This mode is similar to the atrial demand (AAI) mode, except that the ventricle is sensed and paced, rather than the atrium. The refractory period is set at a shorter

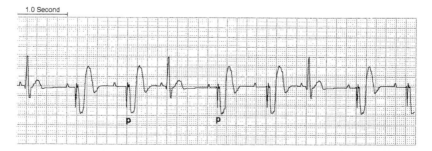

Fig. 3. VVI pacing. The first, fourth, and seventh QRS complexes are native, whereas the others are paced (*p* marks third and fifth beats). Note that in VVI pacing there is no AV synchrony. *From* Chan TC, et al., eds. ECG in Emergency Medicine and Acute Care. Philadelphia: Mosby, 2004; with permission.

interval than in AAI pacing. Because the atrium is not sensed with VVI pacing, AV dissociation or dyssynchrony may occur in patients who have intact atrial function who suffer from AV node blockade, which has disadvantageous hemodynamic and clinical consequences.

DDD pacing

DDD pacing is a form of dual-chambered pacing in which the atria and the ventricles are paced. In DDD pacing the atrium and the ventricle are sensed and paced or inhibited, depending on the native cardiac activity

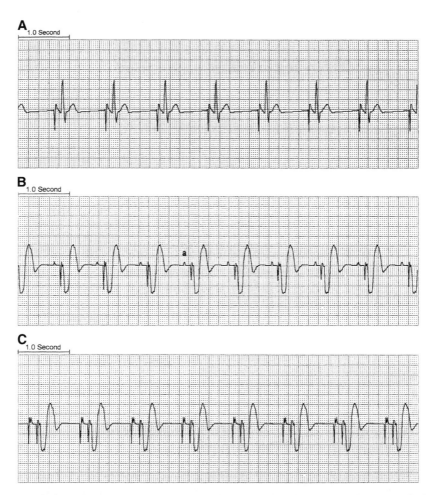

Fig. 4. DDD pacing. (*A*) Atrial pacing with native ventricular QRS activity without ventricular pacing because of intact AV conduction. (*B*) There is atrial sensing of native P waves (*a*) that triggers subsequent ventricular pacing. (*C*) Atrial and ventricular pacing occur. *From* Chan TC, et al., eds. ECG in Emergency Medicine and Acute Care. Philadelphia: Mosby, 2004; with permission.

sensed (Fig. 4). Other forms of dual-chambered pacing are available, such as DVI and VDD, but DDD is the most common. The principle advantage of dual-chambered pacing is that it preserves AV synchrony. Because of this advantage, dual-chambered pacing is increasingly common.

In DDD pacing, if the pacemaker does not sense any native atrial activity after a preset interval, it generates an atrial stimulus (Fig. 4A). An atrial stimulus, whether native or paced, initiates a period known as the AV interval. During the AV interval the atrial channel of the pacemaker is inactive, or refractory. At the end of the present AV interval, if no native ventricular activity is sensed by the ventricular channel, the pacemaker generates a ventricular stimulus (Fig. 4B, C). Following the AV interval, the atrial channel remains refractory during a short, post-ventricular atrial refractory period (PVARP) so as to prevent sensing the ventricular stimulus or resulting retrograde P waves as native atrial activity. The total atrial refractory period (TARP) is the sum of the AV interval and the PVARP. In a simple DDD pacemaker, the TARP determines the upper rate of the pacemaker (upper rate [beats per minute] = 60/TARP).

Mode switching

As one might imagine, if a patient who has a DDD pacemaker were to develop supraventricular tachycardia, the pacemaker might pace the ventricles at the rapid rate based on the atrial stimulus (up to the preprogrammed upper rate limit). To prevent this, most DDD pacemakers now use mode switching algorithms, whereby if a patient develops an atrial tachydysrhythmia, the pacemaker switches to a pacing mode in which there is no atrial tracking, such as VVI. On cessation of the dysrhythmia, the pacemaker reverts to DDD mode, thus restoring AV synchrony without being complicit in the transmission of paroxysmal atrial tachydysrhythmias.

Electrocardiographic findings in the abnormally functioning pacemaker

Abnormal function of pacemakers can be life threatening to patients who are pacemaker-dependent. The 12-lead ECG is an indispensable part of the evaluation of pacemaker function. If there is no pacemaker activity on the ECG, the clinician should attempt to obtain a paced ECG by applying the magnet, which typically switches the pacemaker to asynchronous pacing (a small minority exhibit a different preprogrammed effect or no effect) (Fig. 5). This procedure is useful for assessing pacemaker capture (but not sensing), evaluating battery life, treating pacemaker-mediated tachycardia, and assessing pacemaker function when the native heart rate is greater than the pacing threshold. In the latter case, cautious attempts to slow the rate with maneuvers such as carotid massage, adenosine, or edrophonium administration also can be useful [5]. These should be performed with extreme caution in the pacemaker-dependent patient, however.

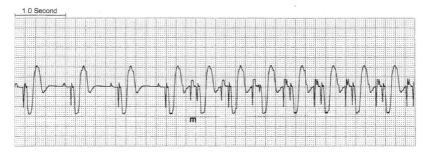

1.0 Second

m

Fig. 5. Effect of magnet application on pacemaker function. Placement of magnet inhibits sensing and reverts the pacemaker to asynchronous pacing. The magnet allows for assessment of capture (but not sensing). In this case, native atrial activity inhibits atrial pacing and triggers ventricular pacing. When the magnet is placed (*m*), atrial sensing is halted and asynchronous atrial and ventricular pacing occurs. The magnet pacing rate is determined by the battery life.

If routine evaluation yields no pacemaker abnormalities and pacemaker malfunction is suspected, the pacemaker should be interrogated by a company technician (this feature is available on most new pacemakers, those with code C or above in position IV of the NASPE/BPEG Generic Pacemaker Code). Many patients carry a card identifying the make and model of pacemaker. If this is not available, inspection of the pacemaker generator on chest radiographs may reveal useful information. Most manufacturers place an identification number in the generator that is visible on chest radiographs. Additionally, chest radiographs may reveal useful information, such as lead dislodgement, migration, or fracture. Causes of abnormal pacemaker function include failure to pace, failure to capture, undersensing, pacemaker-mediated dysrhythmias, pseudomalfunction, and the pacemaker syndrome.

Failure to pace

Pacemaker generator output failure, or failure to pace, occurs when the pacemaker fails to deliver a stimulus in a situation in which pacing should occur. Failure to pace has many causes, including oversensing, pacing lead problems, battery or component failure, and electromagnetic interference (such as from MRI scanning or cellular telephones). Failure to pace manifests on the ECG by an absence of pacemaker spikes at a point at which pacemaker spikes would be expected. In dual-chambered pacing symptoms, isolated atrial or ventricular failure to pace may be evident.

The most common cause of failure to pace is oversensing [6,7]. Oversensing refers to the inappropriate sensing of electrical signals by the pacemaker. Oversensing leads to failure to pace when the inappropriate sensing of electrical signals inhibits the pacemaker from pacing. These abnormal electrical signals may or may not be seen on the ECG.

The most common cause of oversensing is skeletal muscle myopotentials, particularly from the pectoralis and rectus abdominis muscles and the diaphragm [8,9]. In these cases the clinician may be able to reproduce the oversensing by running a 12-lead rhythm strip while having the patient stimulate the rectus and pectoralis muscles. Application of the magnet, which temporarily disables sensing functions, also may be useful. Oversensing caused by skeletal myopotential is almost exclusively a problem encountered in unipolar pacing systems, rather than bipolar pacing systems. Oversensing caused by skeletal myopotentials can be corrected by reprogramming the pacemaker to lower sensitivity or increasing the refractory period.

Oversensing of native cardiac signals also can occur. AV crosstalk occurs, for example, when an atrial sensing system inappropriately senses a QRS complex as native atrial activity. Such oversensing also can be corrected by reprogramming the pacemaker to lower sensitivity of the sensing system or increasing the refractory period. Make-break signals, which are electrical signals produced by intermittent metal-to-metal contact, also can lead to oversensing. Such signals can be caused by lead fracture, dislodgement, or loose connections within the pacemaker generator itself. These lead problems also may cause failure to pace by failing to deliver the pacing stimulus. Battery failure can cause failure to pace, as can primary pacemaker generator failure, although the latter is exceedingly rare. Blunt trauma to the pacing unit can cause failure to pace by damaging the pacemaker or its leads.

Failure to capture

Failure to capture refers to the condition in which a pacing stimulus is generated but fails to trigger myocardial depolarization (Figs. 6–8). On the ECG, failure to capture is identified by the presence of pacing spikes without associated myocardial depolarization, or capture.

Although low current from a failing battery may cause failure to capture as a result of insufficient voltage to trigger depolarization, the most common

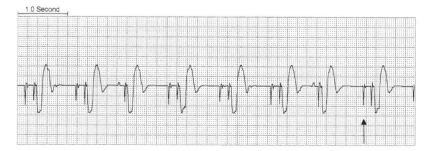

Fig. 6. Failure of atrial capture. Atrial and ventricular pacing spikes are visible, but only the ventricular stimuli are capturing. There are no P waves following the atrial spikes (*arrow*). *From* Chan TC, et al., eds. ECG in Emergency Medicine and Acute Care. Philadelphia: Mosby, 2004; with permission.

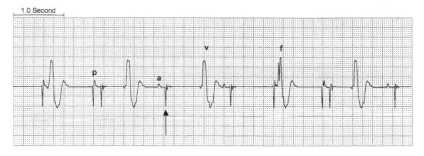

Fig. 7. Failure of ventricular capture. There is intermittent native atrial activity (*a*) and atrial pacing and capture (*p*) when no native activity is present. There is failure of ventricular capture, however, because no QRS complexes following the ventricular pacing spikes (*arrow*). The QRS complexes on this tracing are slow ventricular escape beats (*v*). In the fourth QRS complex, the pacemaker generates a stimulus at the same time a ventricular escape beat occurs, yielding a type of fusion beat (*f*). *From* Chan TC, et al., eds. ECG in Emergency Medicine and Acute Care. Philadelphia: Mosby, 2004; with permission.

cause of failure to capture is elevation in the threshold voltage required for myocardial depolarization, also known as exit block. Exit block can be caused by maturation of tissues at the electrode–myocardium interface in the weeks following implantation [10]. Tissue damage at the electrode–myocardium interface caused by external cardiac defibrillation is another well-known cause of exit block and failure to capture [11]. Some pacemakers are programmed to provide safety pacing with increased pacing output in the setting of abnormal pacemaker functioning or uncertain native activity (Fig. 8).

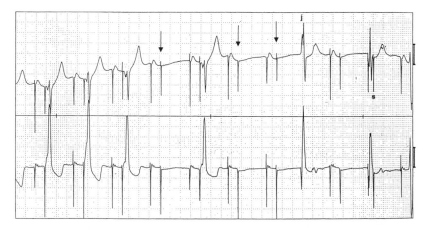

Fig. 8. DDD pacing with intermittent loss of ventricular capture (*arrow*). After the third loss of capture event there is a junctional escape beat (*J*). In the next to last beat, a junctional escape beat is bracketed by two pacing spikes as a form of safety pacing. Rather than inhibiting ventricular pacing (and risk having no ventricular output if the sensed event were not truly a native ventricular depolarization), the AV interval is shortened and a paced output (*S*) occurs.

Undersensing

Undersensing occurs when the pacemaker fails to sense or detect native cardiac activity. At the time of implantation, the pacemaker is programmed to sense cardiac signals of a certain amplitude and frequency given the conditions particular to that individual lead. Anything that changes the amplitude, vector, or frequency of intracardiac electrical signals can result in undersensing. All of the causes for failure to capture also can cause undersensing, as can new bundle branch blocks, premature ventricular contractions (PVCs), or atrial or ventricular tachydysrhythmias. Most cases of undersensing can be remedied by programming the pacing system to a higher sensitivity.

Assessing for the presence of undersensing can be difficult (Figs. 9 and 10). Unlike failure to capture, there is often no obvious finding on ECG to suggest undersensing, because pacing artifacts may or may not be easily detectable. Instead the clinician must infer from the surface ECG whether the pacemaker is sensing properly and responding with an appropriate output based on its program. For example, in patients who have atrial undersensing, the ECG may reveal native P waves that are not being sensed, with resulting atrial pacing spikes (see Fig. 9).

Pacemaker-mediated dysrhythmias

Pacemakers can be useful to treat or prevent dysrhythmias. The pacemaker itself, however, can become a source of dysrhythmias. Examples include pacemaker-mediated tachycardia (PMT), runaway pacemaker, dysrhythmias caused by lead dislodgement, and sensor-induced tachycardias.

Pacemaker-mediated tachycardia

PMT, also known as endless-loop tachycardia, is a re-entry dysrhythmia that can occur in dual-chamber pacemakers with atrial sensing. In contrast

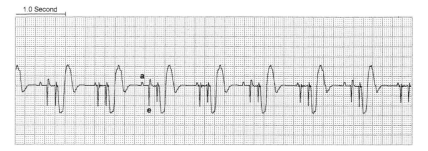

Fig. 9. Atrial undersensing. In this patient with a DDD pacemaker, the native atrial events (*a*) are not sensed. If atrial sensing were occurring, atrial pacing (*e*) would be inhibited. *From* Chan TC, et al., eds. ECG in Emergency Medicine and Acute Care. Philadelphia: Mosby, 2004; with permission.

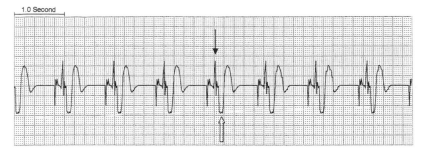

Fig. 10. Ventricular undersensing. In this patient with a DDD pacemaker, intrinsic ventricular events are not sensed. A native, upright, narrow QRS complex (*narrow arrow*) occurs soon after each atrial stimulus, but these complexes are not sensed, and before ventricular repolarization has a chance to get started, ventricular pacing occurs, triggering the wider QRS complexes (*wide arrow*). *From* Chan TC, et al., eds. ECG in Emergency Medicine and Acute Care. Philadelphia: Mosby, 2004; with permission.

to other re-entry dysrhythmias, in PMT the pacemaker itself acts as part of the re-entry circuit.

The atrial channel is programmed with a refractory period (PVARP) immediately after atrial depolarization to prevent sensing of the following ventricular QRS complex or the retrograde P wave that may result from ventricular depolarization. PMT occurs most commonly when a PVC occurs after the PVARP and the atrial channel interprets the resultant retrograde P wave as a native atrial stimulus, which in turn triggers ventricular pacing, which in turn allows the resultant retrograde P wave to again be sensed, and so on. The pacemaker itself acts as the antegrade conductor for the re-entrant rhythm with retrograde VA conduction completing the re-entry circuit loop. It is important to note that PMT cannot exceed the maximum programmed rate of the pacemaker, usually 160–180 bpm. Although a PVC is the most common initiating event, other factors, such as oversensing of skeletal myopotentials or the removal of an applied magnet, also can trigger PMT [12].

On the ECG, PMT appears as a regular, ventricular paced tachycardia at a rate at or less than the maximum upper rate of the pacemaker. Treatment of PMT consists in the application of the magnet, which turns off all sensing and returns the pacemaker to an asynchronous mode of pacing, thus breaking the re-entry circuit. If a magnet is unavailable, PMT can be terminated by achieving VA conduction block with adenosine or vagal maneuvers, which can prolong retrograde and antegrade conduction through the AV node [13–15]. Many modern pacemakers also feature programming to automatically terminate PMT by temporarily prolonging the PVARP or omitting a single ventricular stimulus (Fig. 11).

Runaway pacemaker

The runaway pacemaker is an exceedingly rare phenomenon and represents true primary component failure. The runaway pacemaker consists of

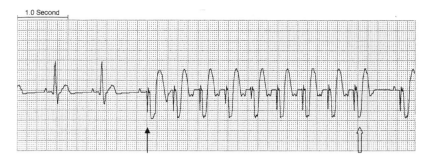

Fig. 11. Pacemaker-mediated tachycardia. The third QRS complex is a paced beat (*narrow arrow*), and causes a retrograde P wave that triggers a run of PMT. In this case the pacemaker detects the PMT and in the penultimate beat (*wide arrow*) temporarily lengthens the PVARP, preventing atrial sensing of the retrograde P wave and breaking the re-entrant loop. *From* Chan TC, et al., eds. ECG in Emergency Medicine and Acute Care. Philadelphia: Mosby, 2004; with permission.

inappropriately rapid discharges at rates of up to 400 pulses per minute, potentially inducing ventricular tachycardia or fibrillation. This phenomenon generally is limited to older generation pacemakers; modern pacemakers have a preprogrammed upper rate limit, which the pacemaker cannot exceed. On the ECG the runaway pacemaker appears as a paced ventricular tachycardia, with a rate often exceeding the expected maximum upper limit of a pacemaker. The runaway pacemaker is a true medical emergency. Application of a magnet may induce a slower pacing rate, and emergency interrogation and reprogramming also may be successful. If this fails, emergent surgical intervention to disconnect or cut the leads is necessary [16].

Dysrhythmias caused by lead dislodgement

A lead that has become dislodged may bounce against the ventricular wall and provoke ventricular extrasystoles or dysrhythmias. Definitive treatment of such cases involves removal or repositioning of the lead.

Sensor-induced tachycardias

Many modern pacemakers are equipped with rate-modulation features that attempt to appropriately increase heart rate to meet physiological demands. This capability is designated by an R in the fourth position of the NASPE/BPEG generic pacemaker code. Examples of types of sensors include ones that respond to vibration, respiratory changes, hemodynamic parameters, and acid–base status. Pacemakers capable of rate-modulation may pace inappropriately if the sensors that regulate the pacemaker are stimulated by nonphysiologic parameters [17]. For example, pacemakers that control rate according to vibration sensors may pace erroneously if they are stimulated by loud noises, vibrations from the environment, or sleeping on the side of the implant [18–21]. Temperature sensors may trigger tachycardia in the febrile patient [22]. Sensors that control rate by monitoring minute ventilation can be triggered by hyperventilation, arm movement, or electrocautery [23,24]. On the ECG, sensor-induced tachycardias appear as paced tachycardias. They are typically benign and cannot exceed the pacemaker's upper rate limit. If needed, they can always be broken with application of the magnet, which returns the system to asynchronous pacing.

Pseudomalfunction

Pseudomalfunction occurs when pacing is actually occurring, but the pacing spikes are not seen. This may happen with bipolar pacing systems and analog ECG recorders, because the voltage in bipolar pacing systems is much smaller than unipolar systems. Pseudomalfunction also occurs when the clinician mistakenly expects the pacemaker to be triggering when it is appropriately inactive.

Rhythms that appear abnormal can occur even when the pacing system is functioning properly. In a DDD pacemaker, AV block rhythms can arise as the native sinus activity increases. As the sinus rate approaches the programmed upper rate limit, the duration of the cardiac cycle, or P-P interval, shortens and becomes less than the TARP. As a result, some native P waves fall within the TARP and go undetected, resulting most commonly in a 2:1 AV block (Fig. 12*A*).

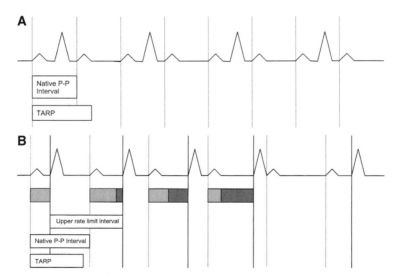

Fig. 12. Pseudomalfunction. AV block schematic for a normally functioning DDD pacemaker. (*A*) Sinus rate increases such that the native P-P interval is shorter than the TARP. Every other P wave occurs within the TARP and the paced QRS complex is dropped, resulting in a 2:1 AV block. (*B*) In this case, the native P-P interval is shorter than the preset upper rate limit interval (minimum cardiac cycle duration for maximum pacemaker rate), but still longer than the TARP. Atrial activity is detected by the pacemaker, but the pacemaker cannot release its ventricular stimulus faster than the upper rate limit resulting in a progressive lengthening of the PR interval until a paced ventricular beat is dropped (Wenckebach).

If the upper rate interval (the cardiac cycle length at the fastest pacemaker rate) is programmed to be longer than the TARP, increased sinus activity actually can lead to a form of Wenckebach rhythm in DDD pacing. This rhythm occurs when the native P-P interval shortens and is less than the upper rate interval but still longer than the TARP. This creates an AV delay as the pacemaker cannot release its ventricular stimulus faster than the upper rate limit allows despite occurring after the TARP. The AV delay increases with successive cycles until a dropped beat occurs, creating a pacemaker-mediated Wenckebach AV block (Fig. 12B). If the atrial rate continues to increase, the P-P interval becomes less than the TARP and a fixed block like that described previously occurs (Fig. 12A).

Pacemaker syndrome

Pacemaker syndrome is a constellation of signs and symptoms in patients who have otherwise normally functioning pacemaker systems resulting from suboptimal pacing modes or programming. The pathophysiology of pacemaker syndrome is complex and multifactorial, but the major factor seems to be suboptimal AV synchrony or AV dyssynchrony [25,26]. This leads to unfavorable hemodynamics and decreased perfusion.

Although the diagnosis cannot be made solely from the ECG, the lack of AV synchrony on an ECG in the appropriate clinical situation suggests the diagnosis. Retrograde P waves suggest VA conduction that in the context of AV dyssynchrony may cause atrial overload, part of the pacemaker syndrome. Additionally, the systolic blood pressure may decrease 20 mm Hg or more when the patient goes from a spontaneous native rhythm to a paced rhythm. Treatment consists in upgrading to dual-chambered pacing to restore AV synchrony.

References

[1] Gregoratos G, Cheitlin MD, Conill A, et al. ACC/AHA guidelines for implantation of cardiac pacemakers and antiarrhythmia devices: executive summary—a report of the American College of Cardiology/American Heart Association Task Force on Practice Guidelines (Committee on Pacemaker Implantation). Circulation 1998;97:1325-35.
[2] Bernstein AD, Camm AJ, Fisher JD, et al. North American Society of Pacing and Electrophysiology policy statement. The NASPE/BPEG Defibrillator Code. Pacing Clin Electrophysiol 1993;16:1776-80.
[3] Sgarbossa EB, Pinski SL, Gates KB, et al. Early electrocardiographic diagnosis of acute myocardial infarction in the presence of ventricular paced rhythm. Am J Cardiol 1996;77:423-4.
[4] Kozlowski FH, Brady WJ, Aufderheide TP, et al. The electrocardiographic diagnosis of acute myocardial infarction in patients with ventricular paced rhythms. Acad Emerg Med 1998;5:52-7.
[5] Atlee JL. Management of patients with pacemakers or ICD devices. In: Atlee JL, editor. Arrhythmias and pacemakers: practical management for anesthesia and critical care medicine. Philadelphia: WB Saunders; 1996. p. 295-329.

[6] Love CJ, Hayes DL. Evaluation of pacemaker malfunction. In: Ellenbogen KA, Kay GN, Wilkoff BL, editors. Clinical cardiac pacing. Philadelphia: WB Saunders; 1995. p. 656–83.

[7] Barold SS, Falkoff MD, Ong LS, et al. Oversensing by single-chamber pacemakers: mechanisms, diagnosis, and treatment. Cardiol Clin 1985;3:565–85.

[8] Secemsky SI, Hauser RG, Denes P, et al. Unipolar sensing abnormalities: incidence and clinical significance of skeletal muscle interference and undersensing in 228 patients. Pacing Clin Electrophysiol 1982;5:10–9.

[9] Gross JN, Platt S, Ritacco R, et al. The clinical relevance of electromyopotential oversensing in current unipolar devices. Pacing Clin Electrophysiol 1992;15:2023–7.

[10] Byrd CL. Management of implant complications. In: Ellenbogen KA, Kay GN, Wilkoff BL, editors. Clinical cardiac pacing. Philadelphia: WB Saunders; 1995. p. 491–522.

[11] Altamura G, Bianconi L, Lo Bianco F, et al. Transthoracic DC shock may represent a serious hazard in pacemaker-dependent patients. Pacing Clin Electrophysiol 1995;18:194–8.

[12] Oseran D, Ausubel K, Klementowicz PT, et al. Spontaneous endless loop tachycardia. Pacing Clin Electrophysiol 1986;9:379–86.

[13] Conti JB, Curtis AB, Hill JA, et al. Termination of pacemaker-mediated tachycardia by adenosine. Clin Cardiol 1994;17:47–8.

[14] Barold SS, Falkoff MD, Ong LS, et al. Pacemaker endless loop tachycardia: termination by simple techniques other than magnet application. Am J Med 1988;85:817–22.

[15] Friart A. Termination of magnet-unresponsive pacemaker endless loop tachycardia by carotid sinus massage [letter]. Am J Med 1989;87:1–2.

[16] Mickley H, Andersen C, Nielsen LH. Runaway pacemaker: a still-existing complication and therapeutic guidelines. Clin Cardiol 1989;12:412–4.

[17] Lau CP, Tai YT, Fong PC, et al. Pacemaker mediated tachycardias in single chamber rate responsive pacing. Pacing Clin Electrophysiol 1990;13:1575–9.

[18] Snoeck J, Beerkhof M, Claeys M, et al. External vibration interference of activity-based rate-responsive pacemakers. Pacing Clin Electrophysiol 1992;15:1841–5.

[19] Gordon RS, O'Dell KB, Low RB, et al. Activity-sensing permanent internal pacemaker dysfunction during helicopter aero-medical transport. Ann Emerg Med 1990;19:1260–3.

[20] French RS, Tillman JG. Pacemaker function during helicopter transport. Ann Emerg Med 1989;18:305–7.

[21] Fromm RE Jr, Taylor DH, Cronin L, et al. The incidence of pacemaker dysfunction during helicopter air medical transport. Am J Emerg Med 1992;10:333–5.

[22] Volosin KJ, O'Connor WH, Fabiszewski R, et al. Pacemaker-mediated tachycardia from a single chamber temperature sensitive pacemaker. Pacing Clin Electrophysiol 1989;12:1596–9.

[23] Vanderheyden M, Timmermans W, Goethals M. Inappropriate rate response in a VVI-R pacemaker. Acta Cardiol 1996;51:545–50.

[24] Seeger W, Kleinert M. An unexpected rate response of a minute-ventilation dependent pacemaker [letter]. Pacing Clin Electrophysiol 1989;12:1707.

[25] Ellenbogen KA, Stambler BS. Pacemaker syndrome. In: Ellenbogen KA, Kay GN, Wilkoff BL, editors. Clinical cardiac pacing. Philadelphia: WB Saunders; 1995. p. 419–31.

[26] Ellenbogen KA, Gilligan DM, Wood MA, et al. The pacemaker syndrome—a matter of definition [editorial]. Am J Cardiol 1997;79:1226–9.

ELSEVIER
SAUNDERS

Emerg Med Clin N Am 24 (2006) 195–208

EMERGENCY
MEDICINE
CLINICS OF
NORTH AMERICA

The Pediatric ECG

Ghazala Q. Sharieff, MD[a,b,*], Sri O. Rao, MD[c]

[a]*Children's Hospital and Health Center/University of California–San Diego,
3020 Children's Way, San Diego, CA 92123*
[b]*Pediatric Emergency Medicine, Palomar-Pomerado Hospitals/California
Emergency Physicians, 555 East Valley Parkway, Escondido, CA 92025, USA*
[c]*Division of Pediatric Cardiology, Children's Hospital and Health Center,
3020 Children's Way, San Diego, CA 92123, USA*

There are many nuances to the pediatric ECG that relate to age-specific changes. These findings relate directly to changes in the myocardium and circulatory system as the individual matures from infancy to adulthood. For example, fetal circulation relies primarily on the right side of the heart and at birth the right ventricle is larger and thicker than the left ventricle. During infancy, increased physiologic stress and work of the left ventricle leads to its enlargement, such that by 6 months it is twice the thickness of the right. By adolescence, the left ventricle is at least 2.5 times as thick as the right [1]. These changes over time lead to the variability of normal ECGs in children, which can sometimes delay interpretation in the emergency department (ED).

A recent review of pediatric ED use reveals that the most common reasons for obtaining ECGs in children are chest pain, suspected dysrhythmia, seizure, syncope, drug exposure, electrical burns, electrolyte abnormalities, and abnormal physical examination findings. Of 71 pediatric ECGs reviewed over a 15-month period, 14 (20%) had clinical significance, such as prolonged QT syndrome, ventricular hypertrophy, or premature ventricular beats [2]. Although a complete review of ECG interpretation is beyond the scope of this article, the authors suggest the use of a systematic approach to ECG interpretation with special attention to rate, rhythm, axis, intervals, ventricular and atrial hypertrophy, and the presence of any ischemia or repolarization abnormalities. This article aids the reader in discerning what is truly essential on the pediatric ECG and also discusses findings in patients with congenital heart disease, hypertrophic cardiomyopathy, and myocarditis.

---

* Corresponding author.
E-mail address: ghazalaqs@hotmail.com (G.Q. Sharieff).

0733-8627/06/$ - see front matter © 2005 Elsevier Inc. All rights reserved.
doi:10.1016/j.emc.2005.08.014   *emed.theclinics.com*

The normal pediatric ECG

There are many systematic techniques for interpreting ECGs and no one method is particularly better than another. A caveat to the electronic interpretation that many ECG machines conduct is that they are manufactured and calibrated with adult values in the software package; hence, the machine interpretation is frequently inaccurate with children. On the other hand, they are reasonably accurate in calculating intervals that are averaged over the entire recording period. The settings of the ECG, however, must be full standard, defined as 10 mm/mV with a standard paper speed of 25 mm/sec. These settings can be changed on the machine to elucidate certain features, but a standard ECG is the only one that should be referenced to normal values. Frequently, additional right ventricular and posterior left ventricular precordial leads (V3R, V4R, and V7) are included with pediatric ECGs to provide additional information on patients who have complex congenital abnormalities. In most pediatric patients, these leads can be ignored.

Table 1 lists the normal pediatric ECG values seen in the newborn, infant, child, and adolescent [3–5]. This table lists normal ranges for heart rate, QRS axis, PR and QRS complex intervals, and R- and S-wave amplitudes, all of which significantly change with age. Rapid changes occur over the first year of life as a result of the dramatic changes in circulation and cardiac physiology. After infancy, subsequent changes are more gradual until late adolescence and adulthood.

Heart rate

In children, cardiac output is determined primarily by heart rate as opposed to stroke volume. With age, the heart rate decreases as the ventricles mature and stroke volume plays a larger role in cardiac output. Age and activity-appropriate heart rates thus must be recognized. Average

Table 1
Pediatric ECG: normal values by age

Age	HR (bpm)	QRS axis (degrees)	PR interval (sec)	QRS interval (sec)	R in V1 (mm)	S in V1 (mm)	R in V6 (mm)	S in V6 (mm)
1st wk	90–160	60–180	0.08–0.15	0.03–0.08	5–26	0–23	0–12	0–10
1–3 wk	100–180	45–160	0.08–0.15	0.03–0.08	3–21	0–16	2–16	0–10
1–2 mo	120–180	30–135	0.08–0.15	0.03–0.08	3–18	0–15	5–21	0–10
3–5 mo	105–185	0–135	0.08–0.15	0.03–0.08	3–20	0–15	6–22	0–10
6–11 mo	110–170	0–135	0.07–0.16	0.03–0.08	2–20	0.5–20	6–23	0–7
1–2 yr	90–165	0–110	0.08–0.16	0.03–0.08	2–18	0.5–21	6–23	0–7
3–4 yr	70–140	0–110	0.09–0.17	0.04–0.08	1–18	0.5–21	4–24	0–5
5–7 yr	65–140	0–110	0.09–0.17	0.04–0.08	0.5–14	0.5–24	4–26	0–4
8–11 yr	60–130	−15–110	0.09–0.17	0.04–0.09	0–14	0.5–25	4–25	0–4
12–15 yr	65–130	−15–110	0.09–0.18	0.04–0.09	0–14	0.5–21	4–25	0–4
>16 yr	50–120	−15–110	0.12–0.20	0.05–0.10	0–14	0.5–23	4–21	0–4

Courtesy of Ra'id Abdullah, MD, University of Chicago, Illinois.

resting heart rate varies with age; newborns can range from 90–160 beats per minute (bpm) and adolescents from 50–120 bpm. The average heart rate peaks about the second month of life and thereafter gradually decreases until adolescence (Fig. 1). Heart rates grossly outside the normal range for age should be scrutinized closely for dysrhythmias.

QRS axis

In utero, blood is shunted away from the lungs by the patent ductus arteriosus, and the right ventricle provides most of the systemic blood flow. As a result, the right ventricle is the dominant chamber in the newborn infant. In the neonate and young infant (up to 2 months), the ECG shows right ventricular dominance and right QRS axis deviation (Fig. 1). Most of the QRS complex is reflective of right ventricular mass. Across the precordium, the QRS complex demonstrates a large amplitude R wave (increased R-/S-wave ratio) in leads V1 and V2, and small amplitude R wave (decreased R-/S-wave ratio) in leads V5 and V6. As the cardiac and circulatory physiology matures, the left ventricle becomes increasingly dominant. Over time, the QRS axis shifts from rightward to a more normal position, and the R-wave amplitude decreases in leads V1 and V2 and increases in leads V5 and V6 (Fig. 2; and see Fig. 1).

PR interval

Similarly, the PR interval also varies with age, gradually increasing with cardiac maturity and increased muscle mass. In neonates, it ranges from 0.08–0.15 sec and in adolescents from 0.120–0.20 sec [3]. The normal shorter PR interval in children must be taken into account when considering the diagnosis of conduction and atrioventricular (AV) block.

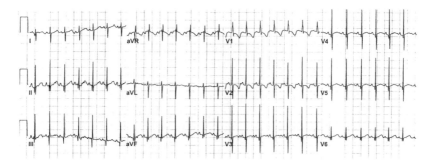

Fig. 1. Normal ECG of 4-week-old infant. The ECG demonstrates right axis deviation and large R-wave amplitude and inverted T waves in the right precordial leads (V1 and V2) indicating right ventricular dominance normally seen in early infancy. Also note the fast heart rate, which is also normal for this age group.

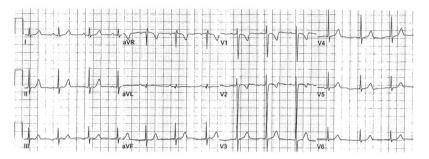

Fig. 2. Persistent juvenile pattern. This ECG in an 11-year-old boy reveals inverted T waves in leads V1 and V2 consistent with juvenile T-wave pattern. Such a finding can persist normally into adolescence.

QRS complex duration

The QRS complex duration varies with age. In children, the QRS complex duration is shorter, possibly because of decreased muscle mass, and gradually increases with age. In neonates it measures 0.030–0.08 sec and in adolescents 0.05–0.10 sec. A QRS complex duration exceeding 0.08 sec in young children (younger than 8 years of age) or exceeding 0.10 sec in older children may be pathologic. As a result, slight prolongation of what may appear as a normal QRS complex can indicate a conduction abnormality or bundle branch block in children.

QT interval

Because the QT interval varies greatly with heart rate, it is usually corrected (QTc), most commonly using Bazett's formula: $QTc = QT/\sqrt{RR}$ interval. During the first half of infancy, the normal QTc is longer than in older children and adults. In the first 6 months of life, the QTc is considered normal at less than 0.49 sec. After infancy, this cutoff is generally 0.44 sec.

T waves

In pediatric patients, T-wave changes on the ECG tend to be nonspecific and are often a source of controversy. What is agreed on is that flat or inverted T waves are normal in the newborn. In fact, the T waves in leads V1 through V3 usually are inverted after the first week of life through the age of 8 years as the so-called "juvenile" T-wave pattern (see Fig. 1). In addition, this pattern can persist into early adolescence (Fig. 2). Upright T waves in V1 after 3 days of age can be a sign of right ventricular hypertrophy (RVH).

Chamber size

An assessment of chamber size is important when analyzing the pediatric ECG for underlying clues to congenital heart abnormalities. P waves greater than 2 mV (2 small boxes) in infants and greater than 3 mV (3 small boxes) in adolescents may indicate right atrial enlargement (RAE). Because the right atrium depolarizes before the left atrium, P-wave duration greater than 0.08 sec (2 small boxes) in infants and 0.12 sec (3 small boxes) in adolescents indicates left atrial enlargement (LAE).

RVH is best seen in leads V1 and V2 with an rSR', QR (no S), or a pure R (no Q or S) wave. RVH also may be suggested by the presence of a large S wave in lead V6, upright T waves in leads V1–V3 after the first week of life, or persistence of the right ventricular dominance pattern of the neonate. Similarly, left ventricular hypertrophy (LVH) is suggested with the presence of tall R waves in lead V6, large S wave in lead V1, left ventricular "strain" pattern in leads V5 and V6, and a mature precordial R-wave progression in the newborn period. Biventricular hypertrophy is seen when ECG criteria for enlargement of both ventricles is seen (Table 2).

The abnormal pediatric ECG

Tachydysrhythmias

The tachydysrhythmias can be classified broadly into those that originate from loci above the AV node (supraventricular), those that originate from the AV node (AV node re-entrant tachycardias), and those that are

Table 2
ECG criteria for ventricular and atrial hypertrophy

Right ventricular hypertrophy
R wave greater than the 98th percentile in lead V1 (see Table 1)[a]
S wave greater than the 98th percentile in lead I or V6 (see Table 1)
RSR' pattern in lead V1, with the R' height being greater than 15 mm in infants younger than 1 year of age or greater than 10 mm in children older than 1 year of age
Q wave in lead V1
Left ventricular hypertrophy
R-wave amplitude greater than 98th percentile in lead V5 or V6 (see Table 1)
R wave less than 5th percentile in lead V1 or V2 (see Table 1)
S-wave amplitude greater than 98th percentile in lead V1 (see Table 1)
Q wave greater than 4 mm in lead V5 or V6
Inverted T wave in lead V6
Right atrial enlargement
Peaked P wave in leads II and V1 that is higher than 3 mm in infants younger than 6 months of age and greater than 2.5 mm in infants older than 6 months of age
Left atrial enlargement
P-wave duration greater than 0.08 seconds in a child younger than 12 months of age or greater than 10 ms in children 1 year and older
P wave minimal or plateau contour
Terminal or deeply inverted P wave in lead V1 or V3R

The presence of any of these is suspicious for hypertrophy. It is not necessary for all of the criteria to be met.
    [a] qR wave pattern in V1 may be seen in 10% of normal newborns.

ventricular in origin. Although AV node re-entrant tachycardias are more common in adults, the vast majority of tachycardias in children are supraventricular in origin. It is important to record continuous ECG or rhythm strips with the child in tachycardia, while medication is being pushed, and when converted to sinus rhythm. On recognition of a tachycardia, stepwise questioning can help clarify the ECG tracing. Is it regular or irregular? Is the QRS complex narrow or wide? Does every P wave result in a single QRS complex?

Sinus tachycardia can be differentiated from other tachycardias by a narrow QRS complex and a P wave that precedes every QRS complex. Sinus tachycardia is a normal rhythm with activity and exercise and can be a normal physiologic response to stresses, such as fever, dehydration, volume loss, anxiety, or pain. Sinus tachycardia that occurs at rest may be a sign of sinus node dysfunction. It is important to keep in mind, however, that the normal range for heart rate is higher in children (see Table 1).

Supraventricular tachycardia (SVT) is the most common symptomatic dysrhythmia in infants and children, with a frequency of 1 in 250–1000 patients [6]. The peak incidence of SVT is during the first 2 months of life. Infants with SVT typically present with nonspecific complaints, such as fussiness, poor feeding, pallor, or lethargy. Older children may complain of chest pain, pounding in their chest, dizziness, shortness of breath, or may demonstrate an altered level of consciousness. The diagnosis often begins in triage with the nurse reporting that "The heart rate is too fast to count."

In newborns and infants with SVT, the heart rate is greater than 220 bpm and can be as fast as 280 bpm, whereas in older children, SVT is defined as a heart rate of more than 180 bpm [7]. On the ECG, supraventricular tachycardia is evidenced by a narrow QRS complex tachycardia without discernible P waves or beat-to-beat variability (Fig. 3). The initial ECG may be normal, however, and a 24-hour rhythm recording (eg, Holter monitor) or an event monitor may be necessary to document the dysrhythmia in cases of intermittent episodes. In children younger than 12 years of age, the most common cause of supraventricular tachycardia is an accessory atrioventricular pathway, whereas in adolescents, AV node re-entry tachycardia becomes more evident [5].

SVT can be associated with Wolff Parkinson White (WPW) syndrome. SVT in WPW syndrome generally is initiated by a premature atrial depolarization that travels to the ventricles by way of the normal atrioventricular pathway, travels retrograde through the accessory pathway, and re-enters the AV node to start a re-entrant type of tachycardia [7,8]. Antegrade conduction through the AV node followed by retrograde conduction through the accessory pathway produces a narrow complex tachycardia (orthodromic tachycardia) and is the most common form of SVT found in WPW syndrome [7,8]. Less commonly re-entry occurs with antegrade conduction through the accessory pathway and retrograde conduction through the AV node (antidromic tachycardia) to produce a wide complex tachycardia [9]. Typical

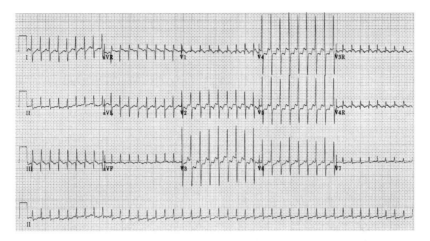

Fig. 3. Supraventricular tachycardia. This ECG demonstrates a supraventricular tachycardia in a neonate. Note the remarkably fast heart rate (260 bpm) and narrow QRS complexes without discernible P waves. It often can be difficult to interpret the ECG in this setting, because the normal QRS complex width is shorter in infants and young children.

ECG findings of WPW are a short PR interval, wide QRS complex, and a positive slurring in the upstroke of the QRS complex, known as a delta wave (Fig. 4). The ECG in most WPW SVT does not show the delta wave, because tachycardia is not conducted down through the accessory pathway. Episodes of SVT in children who have WPW usually occur early in the first year of life [9]. Episodes of SVT often resolve during infancy but may recur later in life, usually from 6–8 years of age [9].

Atrial ectopic tachycardia may be differentiated from SVT by the presence of different P-wave morphologies. Each P wave is conducted to the

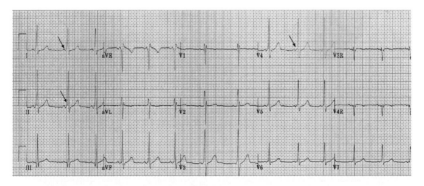

Fig. 4. Wolff Parkinson White syndrome. This ECG is of a 9-year-old boy who presented to the ED with palpitations and minor neck trauma and was found to be in a supraventricular tachycardia. This ECG was done shortly after adenosine was administered and the rhythm converted to sinus. Note the abnormally short PR interval for age and the presence of a delta wave (*arrows*) at the beginning of the QRS complex. The delta wave is not uniformly apparent in all leads.

ventricle, and because the ectopic atrial focus is faster than the SA node, the ectopic determines the ventricular rate (Fig. 5).

Although supraventricular tachycardias are more common than those of ventricular origin, it is important to remember that the normal QRS complex is shorter in duration in children than adults. As a result, a QRS complex width of 0.09 sec may seem normal on the ECG but actually represents an abnormal wide QRS complex tachycardia in an infant. The differential diagnosis of wide complex tachycardia includes sinus/supraventricular tachycardia with bundle branch block or aberrancy, antidromic AV re-entry tachycardia, ventricular tachycardia (VT), or coarse ventricular fibrillation [10]. ECG findings that support the presence of VT include AV dissociation with the ventricular rate exceeding the atrial rate, significantly prolonged QRS complex intervals, and the presence of fusion or capture beats. If there is a right bundle branch block, the presence of VT is supported by a qR complex in V1 and a deep S wave in V6. If there is a left bundle branch block present, then the presence of VT is supported by a notched S wave and an R-wave duration of >0.03 sec in V1 and V2 and a Q wave in V6 [10].

Conduction abnormalities

All degrees of AV block may occur in pediatric patients. It is important to remember that the normal PR interval in infants is shorter and lengthens as cardiac tissue matures with age. A normal appearing PR interval of 0.20 sec may thus in fact represent a pathologic first-degree AV block in an infant or young child.

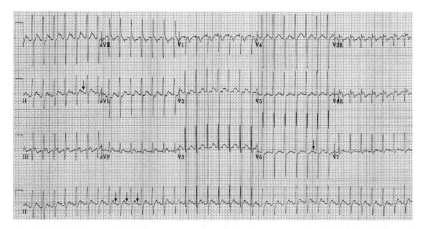

Fig. 5. Atrial ectopic tachycardia. This ECG is of an 18-month-old infant who presented with a several week history of poor feeding and vomiting. The ECG shows atrial ectopic tachycardia. Notice the different P-wave morphologies (*arrows*). Each P wave is conducted to the ventricle, and because the ectopic atrial focus is faster than the sinoatrial node, it determines the ventricular rate.

Complete heart block is a common cause of significant bradycardia in pediatric patients and may be acquired or congenital (Fig. 6). Causes of congenital heart block include structural lesions like L-transposition of the great arteries, or maternal connective tissue disorders. Acquired heart block may result from disorders such as Lyme disease, systemic lupus erythematosus, muscular dystrophies, Kawasaki disease, or rheumatic fever [11].

Bundle branch blocks (BBB) may be present when there is QRS complex prolongation abnormal for a given age. Right BBB occurs with abnormal rightward and anterior terminal forces, frequently manifesting on ECG as an rSR′ pattern in leads V1 and V2. Right BBB is more common than left BBB and can be seen after surgical repair of congenital heart defects, particularly ventricular septal defect repairs. Similarly, left BBB is seen with abnormal leftward and posterior forces, best appreciated in leads V5 and V6. Left BBB is rare in children, however, and the possibility of WPW should be considered, because this syndrome can mimic a left BBB pattern.

Congenital heart

With an incidence of 8/1000 live births, many of the structural congenital heart diseases present in the neonatal period [12]. The signs and symptoms of congenital heart disease may be nonspecific, however. Infants may present with tachypnea, sudden onset of cyanosis or pallor that may worsen with crying, sweating with feeds, lethargy, or failure to thrive [13].

Congenital heart disease lesions that present in the first 2–3 weeks of life are typically the ductal-dependent cardiac lesions. During this period the ductus arteriosus had been sustaining blood flow for these infants. When the ductus closes anatomically at 2–3 weeks of life, these infants suddenly

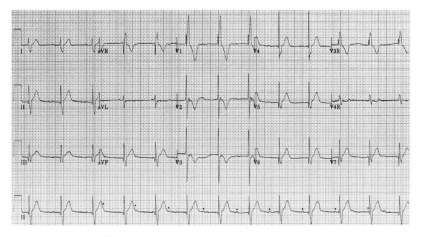

Fig. 6. Complete heart block. The QRS complexes are independent of the P waves (*dots*). This ECG is from a 6-month-old infant who had undergone recent repair of a membranous VSD that temporarily stunned the AV node.

become ill. Depending on the underlying structural abnormality, these neonates present with sudden cyanosis or signs of cardiovascular collapse. These newborns have depended on the ductus arteriosus to supply blood to the lungs—as with tetralogy of Fallot (ToF) or tricuspid atresia (TA)—or to the systemic circulation—as in the case of coarctation of the aorta (CoA) or hypoplastic left heart syndrome (HLHS). The main causes of cyanotic congenital heart disease are ToF, TA, transposition of the great arteries (TGA), truncus arteriosus, total anomalous pulmonary venous return (TAPVR), and pulmonary atresia or stenosis. Time of onset and the common associated ECG findings are listed in Table 3 [14–16].

The other class of congenital cardiac lesions that present in the first month of life are the left-to-right intracardiac shunts, such as ventricular septal or atrioventricular canal defects. As the normal pulmonary vascular resistance falls over the first month of life, any pre-existing left-to-right shunt sees a gradual increase in flow across the shunt, resulting in congestive heart failure. The differential diagnosis of congenital heart diseases that cause congestive heart failure include not only the left-to-right intracardiac

Table 3
Congenital heart abnormalities: time of onset and typical ECG findings

CHD	Onset	RVH	LVH	RAE	LAE	RAD	LAD	RBBB
PDA	2nd–3rd wk		+ (older child)					
ASD	Variable	+		+		+		+
VSD	2nd–12th wk	+	+				+	+
CoA	1st wk	+ (newborn)	+ (older)			+ (newborn)		
ToF	1st–12th wk	+				+		+ (after repair)
TGA	1st wk	+				+	+	
Truncus arteriosis	Variable, infancy	+	+					
Tricuspid atresia	1st–4th wk		+	+			+	
PA	Variable		+					
HLHS	1st wk	+						
AS	Variable		+					
PS	1st–4th wk	+		+		+		
AVC	2nd–3rd wk	+	+	+	+		+	+
HCM	Variable, adulthood		+		+			

AS, aortic stenosis; ASD, atrial septal defect; AVC, atrioventricular canal defects; CoA, coarctation of aorta; HCM, hypertrophic cardiomyopathy; HLHS, hypoplastic left heart syndrome; LAD, left axis deviation; LAE, left atrial enlargement; LVH, left ventricular hypertrophy; PA, pulmonary atresia; PDA, patent ductus arteriosus; PS, pulmonic stenosis; RAD, right axis deviation; RAE, right atrial enlargement; RBBB, right bundle branch block; RVH, right ventricular hypertrophy; TGA, transposition of great vessels; ToF, tetralogy of Fallot; VSD, ventricular septal defect.

shunts, but also HLHS, CoA, TA, endocardial cushion defect, patent ductus arteriosus (PDA), aortic stenosis, interrupted aortic arch, aortic atresia, and mitral valve atresia [17,18].

An ECG should be obtained in all infants suspected of having congenital heart disease. Although the ECG does not make the diagnosis, it can show evidence of conduction abnormalities or chamber enlargement as a result of the congenital defect. In addition, the ECG provides a means of assessing the degree of cardiac flow obstruction, chamber hypertrophy, and the development of dysrhythmias as a result of the congenital heart disease.

Several ECG findings can be associated with specific congenital heart diseases (Table 3). The ECG can seem normal or age-appropriate for some congenital heart diseases. These include cases of PDA, mild-moderate pulmonary stenosis, TGA, ASD, VSD, and CoA, though the presence of abnormalities on the ECG is generally the rule.

RVH is the most common abnormality seen with congenital heart disease and can be seen with pulmonary stenosis, ToF, TGA, and VSD with pulmonary stenosis or pulmonary hypertension, CoA (newborn), pulmonary valve atresia, HLHS, and ASD. RVH may be difficult to distinguish during the early neonatal period because of the normal right ventricular predominance on the ECG at this age. The abnormality becomes clear, however, with later infancy and early childhood.

LVH is seen in lesions with small right ventricles, such as tricuspid atresia, pulmonary atresia with intact ventricular septum, and lesions with left ventricular outflow track obstruction (AS, CoA, hypertrophic cardiomyopathy [HCM]). LVH also can be seen in older children with PDA and larger VSD or AV canal defects (Fig. 7).

In conjunction with ventricular changes, atrial abnormalities can be detected on the ECG with congenital heart disease. RAE occurs with large

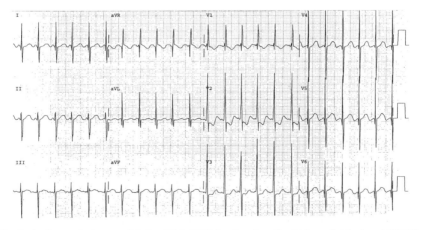

Fig. 7. Atrioventricular canal defect. This ECG is of an 8-week-old boy who had an AVC. The ECG reveals biventricular hypertrophy and left axis deviation not typical for this age group.

left-to-right shunts, causing RA volume overload, and can be seen with ASD, atrioventricular canal defects, tricuspid atresia, Ebstein anomaly, and severe pulmonary stenosis. LAE can be seen with mitral stenosis or insufficiency, left heart obstruction, and complete AV canal defects.

Abnormal QRS axis deviations are seen commonly with congenital heart defects. Right axis deviation can occur with ASD, ToF, CoA, TGA, and pulmonary stenosis. Left axis deviation can be seen with large VSD, tricuspid atresia, TGA, and complete AV canal defects (Fig. 7). Right BBB can be seen with ASD, complete AV defects, small VSD, and after repair of ToF. It is important to keep in mind, however, that incomplete right BBB can be a normal part of the involution of right ventricular forces during infancy and early childhood (Fig. 8).

Hypertrophic cardiomyopathy

Although most cases of HCM are diagnosed at 30–40 years of age, 2% of cases occur in children younger than 5 years of age and 7% occur in children younger than 10 years of age [19]. Clinical presentation varies, with patients experiencing chest pain, palpitations, shortness of breath, syncopal or near syncopal episodes, or sudden death. The hallmark anatomic finding in patients who have HCM is an asymmetric, hypertrophied, nondilated left ventricle with greater involvement of the septum than the ventricular free wall.

ECG findings include LAE and LVH, ST-segment abnormalities, T-wave inversions, Q waves, and diminished or absent R waves in the lateral leads. Premature atrial and ventricular contractions, supraventricular tachycardia, multifocal ventricular dysrhythmias, or new onset atrial fibrillation also may be present.

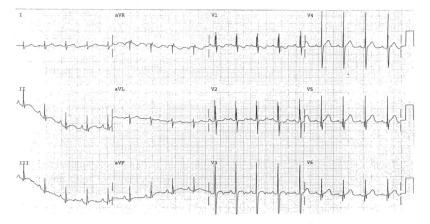

Fig. 8. Incomplete right bundle branch block. This ECG is from a 4-year-old boy. Lead V1 demonstrates an rSR′ pattern, but a relatively narrow QRS complex. The amplitude of the R′ wave approaches criteria for RVH, but this ECG also may be a normal variant.

Myocarditis

An inflammatory condition of the myocardium, this disease has numerous causes; the most common etiology in North America is viral (Coxsackie A and B, ECHO viruses, and influenza viruses) [20,21]. The clinical presentation varies depending on multiple factors, including etiology and patient age. Neonates and infants may present with symptoms such as lethargy, poor feeding, irritability, pallor, fever, and failure to thrive. Symptoms suggestive of heart failure like diaphoresis with feeding, rapid breathing, tachycardia, or respiratory distress also may be present. Older children may complain of weakness and fatigue, particularly on exertion. Signs of poor cardiac function, including signs of congestive heart failure, may be present on examination.

Multiple ECG findings may be present. Sinus tachycardia is the most common dysrhythmia. A tachycardia faster than expected for the degree of fever (10 bpm for each degree of temperature elevation) may indicate myocarditis. Many other dysrhythmias may be associated with myocarditis, including junctional tachycardias, ventricular ectopy, ventricular tachycardias, and even second- and third-degree AV blocks. Morphologically there may be T-wave flattening or inversion and low QRS complex voltage, less than 5 mm in all limb leads.

Summary

Knowledge of the basics of pediatric ECG interpretation is helpful in differentiating normal from abnormal findings. These basics include familiarity with the age-related normal findings in heart rate, intervals, axis and waveform morphologies; an understanding of cardiac physiologic changes associated with age and maturation, particularly the adaptation from right to left ventricular predominance; and a rudimentary understanding of common pediatric dysrhythmias and findings associated with congenital heart diseases.

References

[1] Allen HD, Gutgesell HP, Clark EB, et al, editors. Moss and Adams' heart disease in infants, children, and adolescents. 6th edition. Philadelphia: Lippincott, Williams and Wilkins; 2001.
[2] Horton L, Mosee S, Brenner J. Use of the electrocardiogram in a pediatric emergency department. Arch Pediatr Adolesc Med 1994;148:184–8.
[3] Park MK, Guntheroth WG. How to read pediatric ECGs. 3rd edition. St. Louis: Mosby Year Book; 1992.
[4] Park MK, George R. Pediatric cardiology for practitioners. 4th edition. St. Louis: Mosby; 2002. p. 34–51.
[5] Robinson B, Anisman P, Eshagh E. A primer on pediatric ECGs. Contemp Pediatr 1994;11: 69.
[6] Ziegler VL, Gillette PC, editors. Practical management of pediatric cardiac arrhythmias. Armonk NY: Futura Publishing Co., Inc.; 2001.

[7] Perry JC. Supraventricular tachycardia. In: Garson A Jr, Bricker JT, Fisher DJ, et al, editors. The science and practice of pediatric cardiology. 2nd edition. Baltimore: Williams & Wilkins; 1998.

[8] O'Laughlin MP. Congestive heart failure in children. Pediatr Clin North Am 1999;46(2): 263–73.

[9] Gewitz MH, Vetter VL. Cardiac emergencies. In: Fleisher GR, Ludwig S, editors. Textbook of pediatric emergency medicine. 4th edition. Philadelphia: Lippincott Williams & Williams; 2000.

[10] Silka M. Emergency management of arrhythmias. In: Deal B, Wolff G, Gelband H, editors. Current concepts in diagnosis and management of arrhythmias in infants and children. Armonk NY: Futura Publishing Co.; 1998. p. 319–22.

[11] Fitzmaurice L, Gerardi MJ. Cardiovascular system. In: Gausche-Hill M, Fuchs S, Yamamoto L, editors. The pediatric emergency medicine resource. 4th edition. Sudbury, MA: Jones and Bartlett Publishers; 2004.

[12] McCollough M, Sharieff G. Common complaints in the first month of life. Pediatr Emerg Med Clin N Am 2002;20:27–48.

[13] Savitsky E, Alejos J, Votey S. Emergency department presentations of pediatric congenital heart disease. J Emerg Med 2003;24:239–45.

[14] Woolridge D, Love J. Congenital heart disease in the pediatric emergency department. Pathophysiology and clinical characteristics. Pediatr Emerg Med Reports 2002;7:69–80.

[15] Sharieff G, Wylie T. Pediatric cardiac disorders. J Emerg Med 2004;26:65–79.

[16] Flynn P, Engle M, Ehlers K, et al. Cardiac issues in the pediatric emergency. Pediatr Clin N Am 1992;39:955–83.

[17] DiMaio A, Singh J, et al. The infant with cyanosis in the emergency department. Pediatr Clin N Am 1992;39:987–1006.

[18] al Wigle E. Hypertrophic cardiomyopathy: clinical spectrum and treatment. Circulation 1995;92:1680.

[19] Jouriles N. Pericardial and myocardial disease. In: Marx J, Hockberger R, Walls R, editors. Rosen's emergency medicine concepts and clinical practice. 5th edition. St Louis: Mosby; 2002. p. 1143–4.

[20] Li MM, Klassen TP, Watters LK. Cardiovascular disorders. In: Barkin R, editor. Pediatric emergency medicine, concepts and clinical practice. 2nd edition. St. Louis: Mosby, Inc.; 1997.

[21] Kopeck SL, Gersh BJ. Dilated cardiomyopathy and myocarditis: natural history, etiology, clinical manifestations, and management. Curr Prob Cardiol 1987;12:569–647.

ELSEVIER
SAUNDERS

EMERGENCY
MEDICINE
CLINICS OF
NORTH AMERICA

Emerg Med Clin N Am 24 (2006) 209–225

ECG Techniques and Technologies

J. Lee Garvey, MD

*Chest Pain Evaluation Center and Department of Emergency Medicine,
Carolinas Medical Center, 1000 Blythe Blvd., Charlotte, NC 28203, USA*

Technique of electrocardiographic recording

The electrocardiogram (ECG) continues to be a critical component of the evaluation of patients who have signs and symptoms of emergency cardiac conditions. This tool is now approximately 100 years old [1] and has been a standard in clinical practice for more than half a century. Application of new signal processing techniques and an expansion in the use of additional leads allows clinicians to extract more and more information from the cardiac electrical activity. An understanding of the technology inherent in the recording of ECGs allows one to more fully understand the benefits and limitations of electrocardiography.

As the ECG is a recording of bioelectrical potentials made at the body surface, the interface between the patient's skin and the recording electrodes of the ECG is critical. Much of the artifact introduced into ECG recordings occurs at this junction and is caused by inadequate skin preparation or inadequate skin–electrode contact. Modern ECG electrodes contain a conductive gel that covers the electrode. Optimize the contact of this gel with clean, dry skin. Clip hair and remove superficial dry skin with gentle abrasion before application of adhesive electrodes. Ensure that connections between the electrodes and cables are tight and secure.

The clinical use of ECGs has evolved to include a standard set of 12 leads, providing an array of perspectives to the electrical activity of the heart. Each lead reflects the electrical potential difference measured between two electrodes. These leads are grouped into standard limb leads (I, II, and III), augmented limb leads (aVR, aVL, and aVF), and precordial leads (V1 through V6). The standard bipolar limb leads measure the electrical potential difference (ie, voltage) between electrodes placed at the left arm (as the positive pole) and right arm (as the negative pole) comprising lead I; the left foot (positive) and right arm (negative) for lead II; and the left foot

---

E-mail address: lgarvey@carolinas.org

(positive) and left arm (negative), which form lead III. The electrode placed at the right foot is a ground electrode. Unipolar precordial and limb leads were developed in the 1930s and 1940s as supplements to the standard limb leads. Leads applied to the precordium across the left chest became known as V leads, and those supplemental unipolar electrodes with the exploring (positive) electrode applied to the extremities were termed VR, VL, and VF. The negative pole of the unipolar V leads is termed Wilson's central terminal—an electrical combination of the electrodes applied to the right and left arms and the left leg (Fig. 1). Modification of the central terminal to enhance the amplitude of the unipolar limb leads has resulted in the modern augmented limb leads aVR, aVL, and aVF.

By convention, ECG electrodes are applied at standardized locations on the body. This is required for uniformity in the resulting display of the recordings and to allow comparison of ECGs between individuals and for a single individual over time. It is essential that the ECG electrodes are placed accurately, because malpositioning can reduce the sensitivity in detecting abnormalities or may introduce artifact that may be confused with pathology. Identification of anatomic landmarks by direct palpation is required for accurate and consistent electrode placement. Precordial V leads are placed in the following locations: V1 at the fourth intercostal space (ICS) just to the right of the sternum; V2 at the fourth ICS just to the left of the sternum; V4 at the fifth ICS in the midclavicular line; V3 midway between V2 and V4; V5 and V6 are placed immediately lateral to V4 in the anterior axillary line and midaxillary lines, respectively. These electrodes should be applied to the chest wall beneath the breast in women.

For standard diagnostic resting ECGs, limb lead electrodes are to be placed distally on each extremity and recordings made with the patient

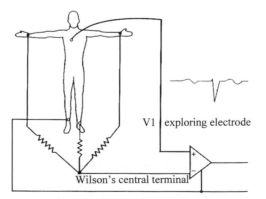

Fig. 1. Schematic for unipolar V lead recording. Wilson's central terminal is (−) pole; exploring (+) pole in this illustration is applied to anterior chest in the V1 position. Wavy lines represent resistors in the connections between the recording electrodes on the three limbs that produce the negative poles for each of the unipolar leads. *From* Wagner GS. Marriott's Practical Electrocardiography, 10th edition. Philadelphia: Lippincott Williams and Wilkins, 2002, with permission.

resting in a supine position. The electrodes should be placed at least distal to the lateral tip of the clavicles and distal to the inguinal lines. Placement in a position too proximal may artifactually distort the ECG, particularly the QRS complex. Again by convention, the electrode wires have been color-coded in a standard manner to help ensure accurate placement by clinical personnel: left arm = black; right arm = white; left leg = red; right leg = green; precordium = brown.

Because placement of electrodes in distal positions on the extremities is impractical for ambulatory patients or those undergoing exercise testing, application of the extremity electrodes more proximally (just inferior to the lateral clavicle tips and midway between the costal margin and the anterior superior iliac spines) helps ensure stability of the electrodes and reduces skeletal muscle artifact. This Mason-Likar [2] system also has been applied to continuous ST segment trend monitoring. It should be noted, however, that nonstandard electrode placement may affect the diagnostic quality of the ECG, but important changes can be identified over the time of the monitoring. Torso limb electrode placement has been noted to effect a rightward shift of the QRS axis, reduction of R-wave amplitude in leads I and aVL, and an increase in R-wave amplitude in leads II, III, and aVF [3].

Instrumentation for ECG recording includes electronic band-pass filters that are designed to minimize artifact while preserving the integrity of the signal. The filters of a typical bedside monitor are optimized for stability of the waveforms and are used routinely for detection of abnormal rhythms. The band-pass filters for such bedside devices in the monitor mode are 0.5–40 Hz. That is, it only allows passage of signals in the range of 0.5 Hz through 40 Hz. A diagnostic electrocardiograph has corresponding filters of 0.05–100 Hz. This band-pass filter is less restrictive and allows more of the inherent signal through. The advantage of the more selective filter of the monitor mode is a reduction in baseline wander caused by respiration and patient movement and the filtering of line noise, typically of 50–60 Hz. Unfortunately the additional filtering of the monitor mode may distort the ST segment by altering the transition at the J point [4]. This may result in the display of the ST segment as elevated or depressed when the ECG recorded using the settings of the diagnostic instrument filters would show the ST segment to be isoelectric, for example. This can result in the over-diagnosis of myocardial ischemia when monitor mode filtering is applied. Obtain a standard, diagnostic ECG using appropriate filtering when entertaining the diagnosis of myocardial ischemia.

ECGs routinely are displayed in columns, first the three limb leads, followed by the three augmented limb leads, and then the precordial leads. Most electrocardiographs record several channels of data concurrently, and vertical alignment of several leads allows accurate identification of the timing of specific components of the waveforms. An alternative display option (the Cabrera sequence) shows leads in a progression corresponding to the anatomic orientation in the six frontal plane leads followed by the six transverse plane or V leads (Fig. 2*A*). The speed at which the paper passes through the printer determines the width of the constituent ECG intervals. Typically, standard paper speed is 25 mm/sec. If specific attention to waveform onset or offset is required, increasing the paper speed to 50 mm/sec displays the ECG in a wider format. Slower paper speeds allow a greater number of cardiac cycles to be visualized on a single print out and are useful in evaluation of rhythm disturbances. At the standard paper speed (25 mm/sec), each 1 mm (small box) corresponds to 40 ms (0.04 sec), and each large box (5 mm) corresponds to 200 ms (0.20 sec). A standard amplitude signal is printed as a reference, with the typical default of 1 mV per cm (Fig. 2*B*). Be sure to verify this when interpreting ECGs, because electrocardiographs automatically adjust the display of the gain to allow large amplitude signals to be completely displayed within the allotted space. For example, large amplitude QRS waveforms associated with left ventricular hypertrophy may

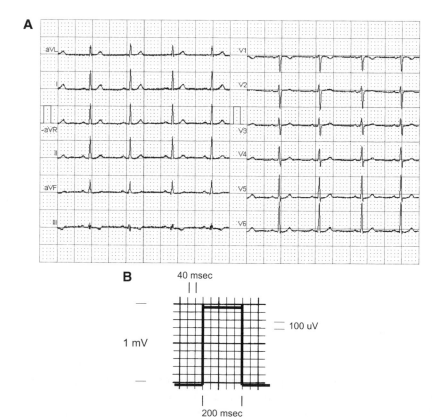

Fig. 2. ECG display formats. (*A*) Cabrera sequence of 12 leads in a single horizontal display. (*B*) Standard ECG amplitude and timing. Square wave marker of voltage amplitude and time notation. Typically ECGs are displayed at a paper speed of 25 mm/sec, corresponding to 40 msec/mm and at 1 mV/cm, corresponding to 100 uV/mm.

cause the gain to be adjusted to 2 mV/cm and ST segment deviations of 0.5 mm would correspond to 100 uV. Alternatively, small amplitude waveforms may be interpreted more easily if the gain is increased to 500 uV/cm.

Technologies enhancing ECGs

Continued advancement of the technology and instrumentation used in recording ECGs has expanded the amount of clinically useful information regarding the electrical activity of the heart that one can now access. Since its development, the ECG has evolved as new technology has become available. With the current expansion of computing methods, processing speed, and signal processing techniques, even more information will be extracted from ECG recordings in the near future. The following discussion illustrates the concept that there is more important information contained within the ECG than is readily apparent by visual inspection of the standard 12-lead ECG.

Atrial leads

Detection of atrial activity and its relationship to ventricular activity are cornerstones of the interpretation of disturbances of cardiac rhythm and conduction. P waves are typically low amplitude signals that may be obscured by other components of the ECG in various pathologic states. P waves are usually identifiable on the standard 12-lead ECG when there is an isoelectric period between the end of one cardiac cycle and the beginning of the next (ie, a T-P interval). If tachycardia or other rhythm disturbance is present, the T-P interval may be obscured and the resulting waveform may include a P wave "buried" within the T wave or other components of the waveform. If atrial activity is initiated after conduction of the impulse from a lower location on the conducting system, an inverted P wave may be inscribed within other parts of the waveform. In these situations, the P waves may be difficult or impossible to identify on the standard 12-lead ECG. Use alternative electrode placement methods when necessary to identify more reliably the presence or absence of such P waves. Noninvasive methods to achieve this detection may include moving the V1 electrode to a position one intercostal space superior (ie, third ICS adjacent to the right sternal border) or reconfiguring recording electrodes to the MCL1 lead or the Lewis lead (Fig. 3). The MCL1 lead is recorded by selecting lead III on the cardiograph and positioning the positive left leg electrode in the V1 position and the left arm electrode in a modified position beneath the left clavicle. The Lewis lead is recorded as lead I of the ECG when modified so that the right arm lead is placed to the right of the manubrium sternum, and the left arm lead is positioned to the right of the sternum in the fifth intercostal space [5]. These strategies orient the leads in positions that are more likely to detect atrial electrical activity.

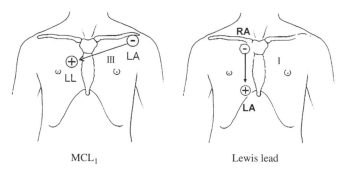

Fig. 3. Modified leads to identify atrial electrical activity. MCL1 lead placement is used to identify atrial activity. Display lead III and move left leg (LL) electrode to the V1 position and the left arm (LA) electrode beneath the left clavicle tip. Lewis lead is recorded as lead I with right arm electrode applied to the right of the manubrium and the left arm electrode applied to the fifth ICS at the right border of the sternum. *Adapted from* Mark JB, Atlas of cardiovascular monitoring. New York: Churchill Livingstone; 1998. p. 136; with permission.

More invasive methods of P-wave detection may be indicated as the clinical situation warrants. Because the atria are anatomically in proximity to the esophagus, placement of an electrode in this position can facilitate identification of atrial electrical activity. An esophageal lead may be constructed using a temporary pacing wire as the exploring electrode. An alligator clip may be required to connect the pacing wire to the V lead cable. When patients have central venous access, use of a saline-filled lumen of the catheter that extends to the proximity of the atrium can facilitate recording of an atrial electrogram (Fig. 4). These leads typically are connected to a V lead cable also. In a direct comparison study, Madias [6] found P-wave amplitude to be greater on recordings made from a saline-filled central catheter than those from a Lewis lead or a lead V1 of the standard ECG.

ST segment monitoring and serial ECGs

In that most conditions requiring emergency cardiac care are dynamic events, the tool used in such investigation should be dynamic also. The typical standard 12-lead ECG records information for a single episode approximately 10 seconds in duration. Contrast this period to the timeframe in which dynamic changes in myocardial oxygen supply and demand change over the course of minutes to hours and the situation in which rhythm disturbances may be manifest literally beat to beat. Bedside monitoring for dysrhythmia detection has been a clinical standard since the 1960s when technology for continuous display of electrocardiographic information became available. Immediate identification and treatment of life-threatening dysrhythmias revolutionized the care of cardiac patients and prompted the development of coronary care units. Similar technologic advances now allow minute-to-minute monitoring intended to detect acute coronary ischemia.

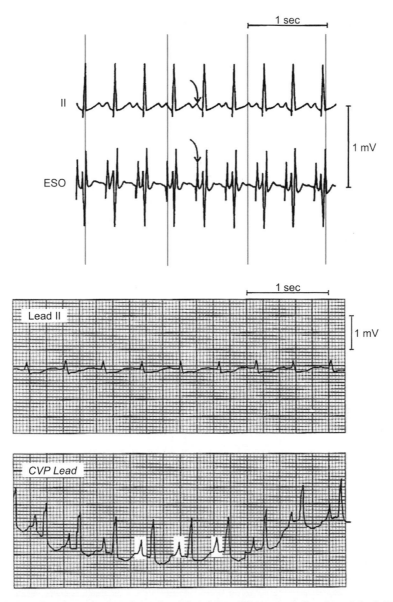

Fig. 4. Invasive electrode detection of atrial activity. (*Upper panel*) Esophageal lead (ESO) demonstrates prominent P waves compared with those recorded using lead II. (*Lower panel*) Atrial activity is displayed prominently (*white boxes*) using a saline-filled central venous pressure catheter (CVP lead) even when surface lead II shows no discernible P wave. *From* Mark JB, Atlas of cardiovascular monitoring. New York: Churchill Livingstone; 1998. p. 136; with permission.

ST segment trend monitoring is the process of dynamic surveillance for cardiac ischemia. ECGs are automatically and repetitively collected by a hardware device [7–9]. Software algorithms analyze the amplitude of the ST segment in each of the constituent standard 12 leads. The ST segment amplitude is plotted over time and displayed. Limits can be set within the device to detect changes automatically in the ST segment amplitude that suggest acute ischemia. Monitors obtain a typical 10-second ECG as often as one or two times per minute and compare the ST segment amplitudes to the initial ECG. This transforms a static snapshot into a dynamic image. Fig. 5 shows an example of an abnormal ST segment trend monitoring session in an individual who presented to the emergency department (ED) with chest pain. This graphical presentation provides a means by which the information from several dozen to several hundred ECGs may be viewed at

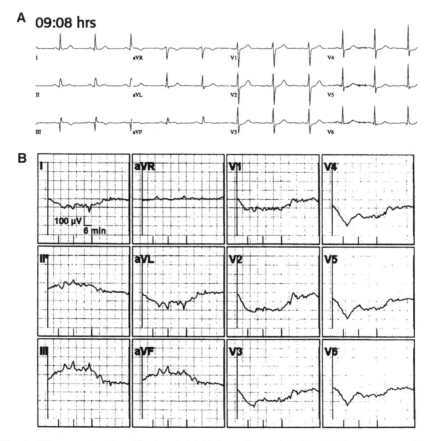

Fig. 5. ST segment trend monitoring. (*A*) Initial nondiagnostic ECG. (*B*) ST segment trending. (*C*) Acute inferior myocardial infarction. (*D*) Coarse ventricular fibrillation. (*E*) Resolution of the significant abnormalities seen above.

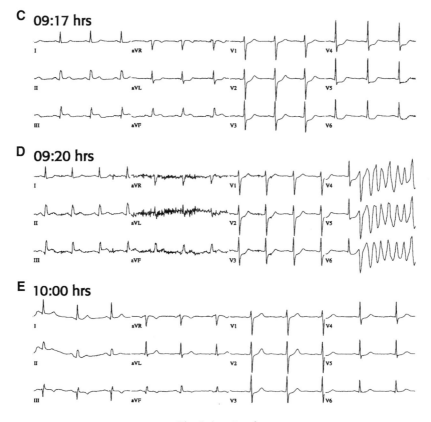

Fig. 5 (*continued*)

a glance. In the case illustrated by Fig. 5, the dynamic changes in the amplitude of the ST segments suggesting acute ischemia and injury precede the initiation of a life-threatening dysrhythmia [7]. This illustrates the concept of dynamic changes associated with acute coronary syndromes and implies that intervention in the early stages (ischemia) would be preferable to detecting only the later, possibly lethal manifestations (ventricular fibrillation). This technique brings the time dimension to the electrocardiogram. The dynamic nature of myocardial ischemia pathophysiology is now matched by real-time monitoring for dynamic electrocardiographic changes.

In a series of 1000 patients, Fesmire [9] showed that ST segment trend monitoring is useful to clinicians in the ED. When compared with the ECG obtained at the time of presentation, ST segment trend monitoring during the ED evaluation improved the sensitivity (34.2 versus 27.5; $P<0.0001$) and specificity (99.4 versus 97.1; $P<0.01$) in detecting acute coronary syndromes. This technique also improved the sensitivity in detecting acute myocardial infarction (68.1 versus 55.4; $P<0.0001$). Diagnostic changes during continuous ST segment monitoring of acute chest pain patients identifies patients for ICU admission, revascularization procedures, and long-term complications [9].

When the instrumentation for continuous ST segment trend monitoring is not available, serial acquisition of standard 12-lead ECGs may be used to monitor for dynamic changes in the ECG. Repeat ECG acquisition should occur when a patient experiences a change in symptoms or if the patient is not responding adequately to therapy. Routinely scheduled repeat ECGs typically are a component of evaluation of the chest pain patient [10]. Access to a patient's previous ECGs assists in the accuracy of interpretation and detection of acute myocardial infarction [11].

Additional leads

Just as continuous ST segment trend monitoring expands the use of diagnostic electrocardiography by enhancing the time-domain, the use of additional electrocardiographic leads enhances the spatial domain addressed by ECGs. The standard 12 leads were not selected or specifically designed to comprehensively address the three-dimensional nature of cardiac electrical activity measurable at the body surface. Consequently some areas of the heart and thorax are suboptimally represented by the standard set of 12 leads. There is no intrinsic reason why the ECG should be limited to 12 leads, and investigators have evaluated the use of additional leads in an attempt to maximize the acquisition of important ECG data. Simple expansions of the standard ECG to include 15 or 18 leads may be done with little or no modification of existing electrocardiographs (Fig. 6). More substantial increases in the array of leads used for electrocardiography and an enhanced system of visual representation of areas of cardiac ischemia/injury incorporate 24–192 leads of data [12–14].

The high lateral and posterior surfaces of the heart are under-represented on the standard 12-lead ECG, making ischemia and injury to these areas more difficult to identify using this tool. In an effort to augment

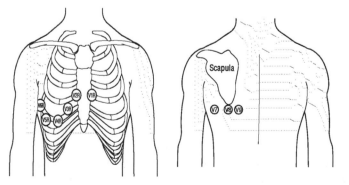

Fig. 6. Additional chest leads. Anatomic location of right chest leads V1R–V6R and posterior chest leads V7–V9.

identification of abnormalities in these geographic regions of the heart, addition of supplementary V leads extending to the posterior left chest have been used [15–18]. These are termed leads V7, V8, and V9, and are positioned at the level of V4–V6 at the posterior axillary line (V7), the inferior border of the scapula (V8), and just to the left of the spine (V9) (Fig. 6). These leads may be used to identify an acute posterior myocardial infarction more readily and to judge more accurately the true extent of the myocardial damage [18].

A more complete description of myocardial injury and additional prognostic and risk stratification information may be provided by the use of additional ECG leads [19,20]. Detection of right ventricle (RV) infarction is often difficult using only standard 12-lead ECGs. By incorporating precordial leads deployed across the right chest, additional views oriented to the right side of the heart are made available. These leads are termed V1R through V6R and are positioned across the right chest in locations corresponding to the V leads of the left chest (Fig. 7). Note that leads V1R and V2R are in the positions of leads V2 and V1, respectively. RV infarction is manifest on ECG when ST segment elevation extends to lead V4R or beyond. Inferior myocardial infarction (IMI) generally is considered to involve less substantial areas of myocardium than anterior myocardial infarction (AMI), and consequently exposes such patients to less risk for adverse outcome than AMI. When RV infarction complicates an IMI, however, patients experience adverse outcomes at a rate comparable to AMI [21]. Zalenski [19] showed that this subgroup of IMI patients at high risk for adverse outcome can be identified by attention to ST segment elevation in lead V4R.

Although the anatomic location of the right ventricle beneath the sternum potentially exposes it to injury as a result of blunt trauma, findings

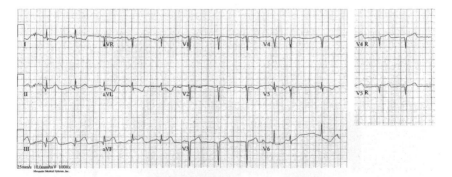

Fig. 7. Inferior myocardial infarction complicated by right ventricular involvement. ST segment elevation in inferior leads (leads III and aVF, greater than lead II, suggesting right coronary artery lesion) is accompanied by reciprocal ST segment depression in leads aVL and I. There is also evidence of an old anterior infarction. Note the subtle ST segment elevation in leads V4R and V5R, indicating right ventricular involvement.

in lead V4R was not found to add substantially to the evaluation of trauma patients when compared with the standard ECG [22].

Because the standard 12-lead ECG has poor sensitivity in detecting acute coronary syndromes at the time of presentation, more extensive arrays of electrodes have been used in an attempt to enhance the detection of ischemia and infarction [12,14,23]. Criteria for diagnosis of abnormalities using these systems may be complicated or may involve subjective interpretation of the results. To assist with this, an automated interpretation algorithm has been incorporated into an 80-lead system for interpretation of the body surface map of isopotentials [13]. In this system, an anterior harness containing 64 electrodes and a posterior harness containing 16 electrodes record unipolar ECGs referenced to Wilson's central terminal. Isopotential maps are constructed using the potential at each electrode site at the J point or at the J + 60 msec point (Fig. 8). Abnormalities in the isopotential map may indicate ischemia or infarction even when the standard 12-lead ECG is nondiagnostic (Fig. 9).

QT dispersion

The QT interval encompasses ventricular depolarization and repolarization. Measurement of this interval is a standard component of ECG analysis. It has been noted that the QT interval varies between the leads of the standard ECG, and this dispersion has been interpreted to reflect an inhomogeneity of repolarization. The measurement of this QT dispersion interval (QTd—the difference between the longest and shortest QT interval on a 12-lead ECG) often is complicated by difficulty in determining the exact end of the T wave, the endpoint for the QT interval. Abnormal dispersion of repolarization is suggested to increase risk for dysrhythmia and may be associated with acute myocardial ischemia [24,25]. This explanation for QTd, however, has generated significant controversy [26–28]. A wide range in QTd values has been reported in healthy subjects (range, 10–71 msec), and even though most studies find prolonged QTd values for cardiac patients, the differentiation between normal and abnormal QTd is often

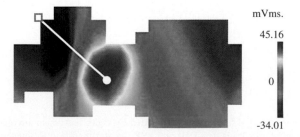

Fig. 8. Body surface map. Electrode array of 64 anterior leads and 16 posterior leads and isopotential map. Diagnostic algorithm interpretation statements are included in this device's report.

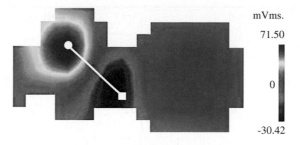

mVms.

71.50

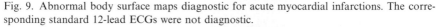

0

-30.42

Fig. 9. Abnormal body surface maps diagnostic for acute myocardial infarctions. The corresponding standard 12-lead ECGs were not diagnostic.

difficult [28]. Malik suggests that only grossly abnormal values for QTd (eg, ≥ 100 msec) are outside the range of measurement error and may identify grossly abnormal repolarization [28]. It is now believed that abnormal QTd most likely represents abnormality of the T-wave loop [29–31]. This interval ultimately may prove useful in assisting in the diagnosis of acute coronary artery disease, as evidenced by its potential as an aid in the evaluation of exercise stress testing [32].

High frequency ECGs

The standard ECG displays waveforms within the 0.05–100 Hz portion of the spectrum. Signals that represent higher frequencies within the ECG routinely are excluded from presentation and analysis. This exclusion was decided on because such high frequency components (> 100 Hz) are typically of low amplitude and are difficult to differentiate from electrical noise. High frequency, low amplitude signals, however, have been identified within the QRS complex and possibly are markers of abnormal conduction associated with cardiac pathology [33–35]. Recent advances in signal acquisition and digital signal processing allow high frequency components (HFECGs) to be recorded up to 250 Hz. To make reliable recordings of these components, more rapid data sampling (1000 samples/sec) is required. Digital signal averaging is used in HFECGs to differentiate the low amplitude HF signals from background noise. Signal averaging is a technique of electronically averaging recordings from many cardiac cycles and results in the generation of composite waveforms for the electrocardiographic leads. Up to 100 or more cardiac cycles are averaged in a process to enhance the signal-to-noise ratio. Fig. 10 shows HFECGs recorded using standard lead placement. Abnormal HF components are identified when a reduced amplitude zone (RAZ) is seen within the waveform recorded in the 150–250 Hz range. The definition of an abnormal HFECG incorporates the spatial grouping and magnitude of the RAZs [35]. Abnormal HFECGs may identify patients with heart disease [35,36] (eg, congestive heart failure, coronary artery disease), though their resting 12-lead ECG seems normal [37]. The use of this technology in the clinical

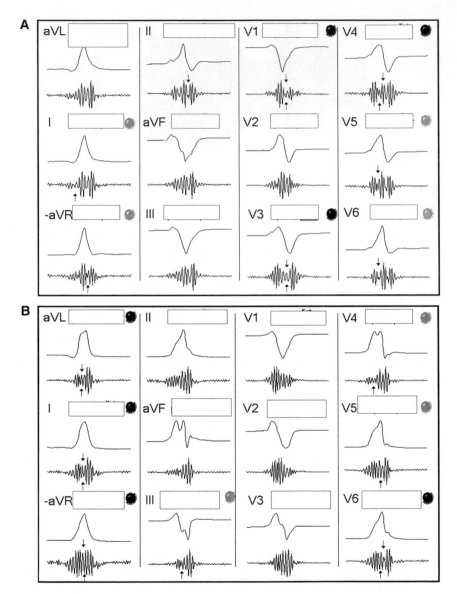

Fig. 10. High frequency ECGs. (*A*) Normal HFECG. Though a few leads have detectable re-duced amplitude zones (RAZs, indicated by *arrows*) within the QRS complexes, they are not of sufficient magnitude or spatial orientation to meet the definition for abnormal HFECG. (*B*) Ab-normal HFECG with reduced amplitude zones (RAZs). *Dark circles* to the right of the leads indicate abnormal RAZ. (*C*) Standard ECG was normal in the patient with an abnormal HFECG (presented in *B*) who was experiencing myocardial ischemia.

C

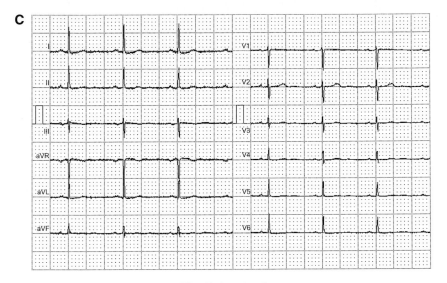

Fig. 10 (*continued*)

setting is now feasible because of real-time acquisition and interpretation of data facilitated by modern computing methods.

References

[1] Burch GE, DePasquale NP. A history of electrocardiography. San Francisco: Norman Publishing; 1990.

[2] Mason RE, Likar I. A new system of multiple-lead exercise electrocardiography. Am Heart J 1966;71:196–205.

[3] Papouchado M, Walker PR, James MA, et al. Fundamental differences between the standard 12-lead electrocardiograph and the modified (Mason-Likar) exercise lead system. Am J Emerg Med 1987;8:725–33.

[4] Mark JB. Atlas of cardiovascular monitoring. New York: Churchill Livingstone; 1998.

[5] Constant J. Learning electrocardiography. 3rd edition. Boston: Little Brown and Co.; 1987.

[6] Madias JE. Comparison of P waves recorded on the standard electrocardiogram, the "Lewis lead," and "saline-filled central venous catheter"-based, intracardiac electrocardiogram. Am J Cardiol 2004;94:474–8.

[7] Velez J, Brady WJ, Perron AD, et al. Serial electrocardiography. Am J Emerg Med 2002;20: 43–9.

[8] Drew BJ, Krucoff MW. Multilead ST-segment monitoring in patients with acute coronary syndromes: a consensus statement for healthcare professionals. ST-Segment Monitoring Practice Guideline International Working Group. Am J Crit Care 1999;8:372–86.

[9] Fesmire FM, Percy RF, Bardoner JB, et al. Usefulness of automated serial 12-lead ECG monitoring during the initial emergency department evaluation of patients with chest pain. Ann Emerg Med 1998;31:3–11.

[10] ACEP Clinical Policy. Critical issues in the evaluation and management of adult patients presenting with suspected acute myocardial infarction or unstable angina. Ann Emerg Med 2000;35:521–44.

[11] Ohlsson M, Ohlin H, Wallerstedt SM, et al. Usefulness of serial electrocardiograms for diagnosis of acute myocardial infarction. Am J Cardiol 2001;88:478–81.

[12] Pahlm-Webb U, Pahlm O, Sadanandan S, et al. A new method for using the direction of ST-segment deviation to localize the site of acute coronary occlusion: the 24-view standard electrocardiogram. Am J Med 2002;113:75–8.

[13] McClelland AJ, Owens CG, Menown IB, et al. Comparison of the 80-lead body surface map to physician and to 12-lead electrocardiogram in detection of acute myocardial infarction. Am J Cardiol 2003;92:252–7.

[14] Wung SF, Lux RL, Drew BJ. Thoracic location of the lead with maximal ST-segment deviation during posterior and right ventricular ischemia: comparison of 18-lead ECG with 192 estimated body surface leads. J Electrocardiol 2000;33(Suppl):167–74.

[15] Matetzky S, Freimark D, Feinberg MS, et al. Acute myocardial infarction with isolated ST-segment elevation in posterior chest leads V7–9: "hidden" ST-segment elevations revealing acute posterior infarction. J Am Col Cardiol 1999;34:748–53.

[16] Agarwal JB, Khaw K, Aurignac F, et al. Importance of posterior chest leads in patients with suspected myocardial infarction, but nondiagnostic, routine 12-lead electrocardiogram. Am J Cardiol 1999;83:323–6.

[17] Brady WJ, Erling B, Pollack M, et al. Electrocardiographic manifestations: acute posterior wall myocardial infarction. J Emerg Med 2001;20:391–401.

[18] Somers MP, Brady WJ, Bateman DC, et al. Additional electrocardiographic leads in the ED chest pain patient: right ventricular and posterior leads. Am J Emerg Med 2003;21:563–73.

[19] Zalenski RJ, Rydman RJ, Sloan EP, et al. ST segment elevation and the prediction of hospital life-threatening complications: the role of right ventricular and posterior leads. J Electrocardiol 1998;31(Suppl):164–71.

[20] Brady WJ, Hwang V, Sullivan R, et al. a comparison of 12- and 15-lead ECGs in ED chest pain patients: impact on diagnosis, therapy, and disposition. Am J Emerg Med 2000;18:239–43.

[21] Zehender M, Kasper W, Kauder E, et al. Right ventricular infarction as an independent predictor of prognosis after acute inferior myocardial infarction. N Engl J Med 1993;328:981–8.

[22] Walsh P, Marks G, Aranguri C, et al. Use of V4R in patients who sustain blunt chest trauma. J Trauma 2001;51:60–3.

[23] Horacek BM, Wagner GS. Electrocardiographic ST-segment changes during acute myocardial ischemia. Card Electrophysiol Rev 2002;6:196–203.

[24] Zareba W, Moss AJ, le Cessie S. Dispersion of ventricular repolarization and arrhythmic cardiac death in coronary artery disease. Am J Cardiol 1994;74:550–3.

[25] Sportson SC, Taggart P, Sutton PM, et al. acute ischemia: a dynamic influence on QT dispersion. Lancet 1997;349:306–9.

[26] Malik M, Camm AJ. Mystery of QTc interval dispersion. Am J Cardiol 1997;79:785–7.

[27] Rautaharju PM. QT and dispersion of ventricular repolarization: the greatest fallacy in electrocardiography in the 1990s. Circulation 1999;99:2477–8.

[28] Malik M, Batchvarov VN. Measurement, interpretation and clinical potential of QT dispersion. J Am Coll Cardiol 2000;36:1749–66.

[29] Lee KW, Kligfield P, Dower GE, et al. QT dispersion, T-wave projection, and heterogeneity of repolarization in patients with coronary artery disease. Am J Cardiol 2001;87:148–51.

[30] Somberg JC, Molnar J. Usefulness of QT dispersion as an electrocardiographically derived index [comment, review]. Am J Cardiol 2002;89:291–4.

[31] Kautzner J. QT interval measurements. Card Electrophysiol Rev 2002;6:273–7.

[32] Koide Y, Yotsukura M, Yoshino H, et al. Usefulness of QT dispersion immediately after exercise as an indicator of coronary stenosis independent of gender or exercise-induced ST-segment depression. Am J Cardiol 2000;86:1312–7.

[33] Abboud S, Cohen J, Selwyn A, et al. Detection of transient myocardial ischemia by computer analysis of standard and signal-averaged high-frequency electrocardiograms in patients undergoing percutaneous transluminal coronary angioplasty. Circulation 1987;76:585–96.

[34] Abboud S. High-frequency electrocardiogram analysis of the entire QRS in the diagnosis and assessment of coronary artery disease. Prog Cardiovasc Dis 1993;35:311–28.

[35] Schlege TT, Kulecz WB, DePalma JL, et al. Real-time 12-lead high-frequency QRS electrocardiography for enhanced detection of myocardial ischemia and coronary artery disease. Mayo Clin Proc 2004;79:339–50.

[36] Pettersson J, Pahlm O, Carro E, et al. Changes in high-frequency QRS components are more sensitive than ST-segment deviation for detecting acute coronary artery occlusion. J Am Coll Cardiol 2000;36:1827–34.

[37] Abboud S, Belhassen B, Miller HI, et al. High frequency electrocardiography using an advanced method of signal averaging for non-invasive detection of coronary artery disease in patients with normal conventional electrocardiogram. J Electrocardiol 1986;19:371–80.

ELSEVIER
SAUNDERS

Emerg Med Clin N Am 24 (2006) 227–235

EMERGENCY
MEDICINE
CLINICS OF
NORTH AMERICA

Electrode Misconnection, Misplacement, and Artifact

Richard A. Harrigan, MD

Department of Emergency Medicine, Temple University School of Medicine, Jones Hall,
Room 1005, Park Avenue and Ontario Street, Philadelphia, PA 19140, USA

The emergency physician (EP) examines the electrocardiogram (ECG) looking for evidence of normalcy and for signs of ischemia, dysrhythmia, and many other variations of normal, such as are described in this issue. An under appreciated cause of ECG abnormality is electrode misconnection and misplacement. This occurs when the ECG electrode is mistakenly connected to the wrong part of the body (electrode misconnection, as can occur most commonly with the limb electrodes, I, II, III, aVR, aVL, and aVF) or is placed improperly on the body (electrode misplacement, such as can occur most easily with the precordial electrodes, V1–V6). Knowledge of the common patterns of electrode misconnection and misplacement lead to the ready recognition of this phenomenon in everyday practice.

Using recordings from four limb electrodes (RA or right arm, LA or left arm, RL or right leg, and LL or left leg), six frontal plane electrocardiographic tracings, or leads, are generated. An understanding of limb electrode misconnection begins with a review of the derivation of the three limb leads (I, II, and III) and the three augmented leads (aVR, aVL, and aVF) (Fig. 1). In the horizontal plane, six precordial electrodes (V1–V6) yield six electrocardiographic leads (V1–V6); although they too can be misconnected, the pitfalls of right/left and arm/leg reversal do not apply here. Recording problems with the precordial electrodes more significantly are caused by improper positioning of the individual electrodes on the body surface because of anatomic variation. Common examples of limb electrode reversal and precordial electrode misconnection and misplacement are described.

E-mail address: richard.harrigan@tuhs.temple.edu

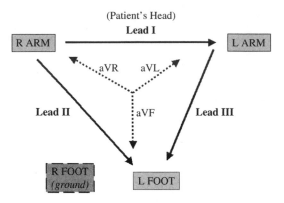

Fig. 1. The standard limb and augmented leads on the 12-lead ECG. Solid arrows represent leads I (RA→LA), II (RA→LL), and III (LA→LL), where RA = right arm, LA = left arm, and LL = left leg. *Dotted arrows* depict leads aVR, aVL, and aVF. *Arrowheads* are located at the positive pole of each of these vectors. The right leg serves as a ground electrode, and as such is not directly reflected in any of the six standard and augmented lead tracings.

Limb electrode misconnection

There are myriad possible ways to misconnect the four limb electrodes when recording the 12-lead ECG; commonly, such errors result from reversal of right/left or arm/leg. Common limb electrode reversals therefore include the following: RA/LA, RL/LL, RA/RL, and LA/LL. More bizarre reversals involving reversal of right/left and arm/leg also yield predictable changes, but are intuitively less likely to occur, because they require, by definition, two operator errors. Only the four common limb electrode reversals thus are discussed in detail, followed by those less common misconnections (RA/LL and LA/RL).

Arm electrode reversal (RA/LA)

Fortuitously, this is the most common limb electrode misconnection and one of the easiest to detect [1–4]. Because the RA and LA electrodes are reversed, lead I is reversed, resulting in an upside-down representation of the patient's normal lead I tracing (Fig. 2; and see Fig. 1). Lead I thus features, in most cases, an inverted P-QRS-T, yielding most saliently a rightward QRS axis deviation (given the predominant QRS vector is negative in lead I and positive in lead aVF) or an extreme QRS axis deviation (predominant QRS vector is negative in leads I and aVF). Furthermore, an inverted P wave in lead I is distinctly abnormal and should prompt the EP to consider limb electrode misconnection, dextrocardia, congenital heart disease, junctional rhythm, or ectopic atrial rhythm. Reversal of the arm electrodes means reversal of the waveforms seen in leads aVR and aVL—thus the EP may see a normal appearing, or upright, P-QRS-T in lead aVR. This too is distinctly unusual, because the major vector of cardiac depolarization

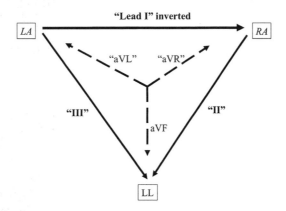

Fig. 2. Schematic of RA/LA electrode reversal. Reversal of the arm electrodes (shown in italics) affects leads I, II, and III, and leads aVR and aVL. Affected leads are shown in quotation marks in this and subsequent schematic Figs. and are shown as they appear on the tracing, ie, in the lead II position on the tracing, lead III actually appears (and vice versa).

usually is directed leftward and inferiorly, or away from, the positive pole of lead aVR, which is oriented rightward and superiorly (see Fig. 1). One final clue to arm electrode reversal is to compare the major QRS vector of leads I and V6. Both are normally directed in roughly the same direction, because both reflect vector activity toward the left side of the heart. Disparity between these two leads' predominant QRS deflection should prompt the EP to consider limb electrode reversal (Fig. 3).

Electrode reversals involving the right leg

The right leg electrode (see Fig. 1) serves as a ground and as such does not contribute directly to any individual lead [5,6]. There is virtually no potential difference between the two leg electrodes, thus inadvertent leg electrode reversal (RL/LL) results in no distinguishable change in the 12-lead ECG. Moving the right leg electrode to a location other than the left leg causes a disturbance in the amplitude and the morphology of the complexes seen in the limb leads [3]. Electrode reversals involving other misconnections of the right leg electrode (RA/RL and LA/RL) can be considered together because of a telltale change attributable to reversals involving the right leg: the key to recognizing these misconnections is recalling that they result in one of the standard leads (I, II, or III) displaying nearly a flat line [5,6]. The location of the flat line depends on the lead misconnection and hinges on the fact that the ECG views the right leg electrode as a ground with no potential difference between the right and left legs [3]. In RA/RL reversal, the lead II vector, usually RA→LL, is now *RL*→LL, and thus a flat line appears in lead II (Figs. 4 and 5). Similarly, LA/RL reversal results in a flat line along the lead III vector, which is now bounded by *RL* and LL electrodes, rather than the normal LA and LL electrodes (Fig. 6).

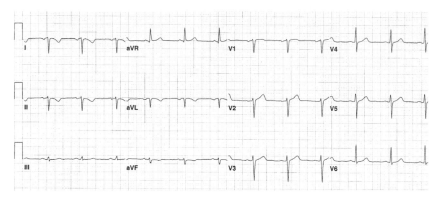

Fig. 3. RA/LA electrode reversal. Note the characteristic changes in this most common lead reversal. Lead I features an upside-down P-QRS-T, and the major vector of its QRS complex is uncharacteristically opposite to that seen in lead V6. The waveforms in lead aVR appear normal and are actually those that appear in aVL when the electrodes are placed properly. Leads II and III also are reversed, which in this tracing yields a principally negative vector in lead II; this is also unusual.

Left arm/left leg electrode reversal

Misconnection of the left-sided electrodes (LA and LL) is the most difficult limb electrode reversal to detect [3,7]. An ECG with LA/LL electrode misconnection usually appears normal and may not be suspected until compared with an old ECG. Making matters worse, the variability between old and new tracings may be ascribed to underlying patient disease, such as cardiac ischemia, if LA/LL electrode reversal is not considered. What makes LA/LL electrode reversal so difficult to detect is that the changes that ensue

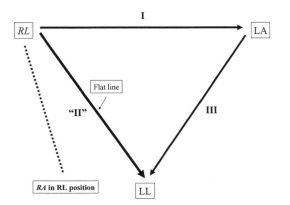

Fig. 4. Schematic of RA/RL electrode reversal. Reversal of the right-sided electrodes (shown in italics) allows lead II (linking the RA and LL normally, but now linking RL and LL because of the misconnection) to demonstrate the lack of potential difference between the leg electrodes. Lead II thus features a flat line.

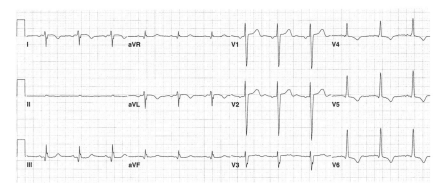

Fig. 5. RA/RL electrode reversal. The classic finding of an electrode misconnection involving the right leg is seen in lead II, in which the tracing is nearly flat line, or isoelectric. Because lead II normally depicts the RA→LL vector and a flat line results from the no potential difference between the leg electrodes, the RL electrode must be in the RA position (see Fig. 4). The other limb leads feature morphologic and amplitude changes from the patient's baseline, but these need not be remembered; the key is recognition of the flat line in lead II.

occur somewhat in parallel; that is, two inferior leads (II and aVF) become lateral (I and aVL, respectively), and vice versa (Fig. 7). Lead III is inverted, but the major QRS vector of lead III may be principally positive or principally negative in normal conditions, so this is not a red flag. Further obscuring this lead misconnection, lead aVR remains unaffected (Fig. 8).

Attention to the P-wave amplitude in leads I and II and P-wave morphology in lead III has been advanced as a means to detect LA/LL electrode misconnection. Normally the P wave in lead II is larger than that seen in lead I, because the normal P axis vector is between +45° and +60°, similar to the

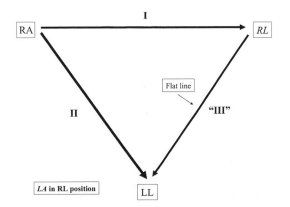

Fig. 6. Schematic of LA/RL electrode reversal. Reversal of the LA and RL electrodes (shown in italics) allows lead III (linking the LA and LL normally, but now linking RL and LL because of the misconnection) to demonstrate the lack of potential difference between the leg electrodes. Lead III thus features a flat line.

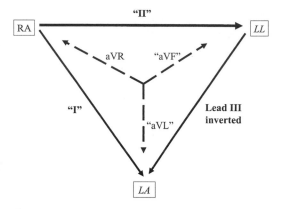

Fig. 7. Schematic of LA/LL electrode reversal. Reversal of the two left-sided electrodes (shown in italics) leads to the appearance of an inverted lead III. Furthermore, leads I and II are reversed, as are leads aVL and aVF. This results in two lateral leads (I and aVL) reversing with two inferior leads (II and aVF, respectively). Lead aVR remains unaffected. These changes result in an LA/LL reversal being the most difficult electrode reversal to detect.

vector of lead II (+60°). With LA/LL reversal, however, the P wave is usually larger in lead I than in lead II, and thus serves as a hint even before looking at an old tracing. Furthermore, if a biphasic P wave appears in lead III, the second portion normally is deflected negatively; thus, if the terminal portion is positive, this too serves as a hint to LA/LL electrode reversal. Using these two features, reversal of LA and LL electrodes was detected in 90% of 70 cases in one report [7]. Tracings demonstrating atrial flutter make LA/LL electrode misconnection easier to detect, because the flutter waves—usually most salient in the inferior leads II, III, and aVF—would now appear most prominently in leads I, aVL, and III. Atrial fibrillation obviously would make LA/LL electrode reversal impossible to detect by P-wave or flutter wave characteristics [3,7].

Other less common limb electrode reversals

Misconnection of other limb electrodes (eg, RA/LL and both arms/both legs) involve multiple operator errors and thus are encountered less often. RA/LL reversal is easy to recognize, because upside-down P-QRS-T complexes appear in all leads except aVL, which is unaffected. Lead aVR thus appears normal—another hallmark of lead misconnection. Placing both leg electrodes on the arms but maintaining sidedness is best recognized by the flat line that appears in lead I—again, misplacement of the RL electrode to anywhere but the LL results in a near isoelectric appearance of the lead that connects the misplaced RL and LL electrodes. This occurs because that lead is showing no potential difference between the RL and LL electrodes, which have been misplaced on the arms (lead I position) [3].

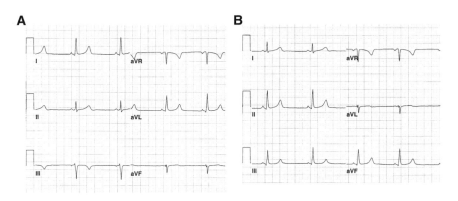

Fig. 8. LA/LL electrode reversal. Limb leads only are shown here from the same patient at two points in time. (*A*) LA/LL electrode reversal. (*B*) Tracing performed after the electrodes were repositioned correctly in this patient undergoing an ED evaluation for chest pain. Comparing (*A*) and (*B*), note that lead III is inverted, and the two other inferior leads (II and aVF) are actually the lateral leads (I and aVL, respectively), and vice versa. Scrutiny of the P wave in lead I suggests LA/LL misconnection in (*A*), because the amplitude of the P wave is larger in lead I than in lead II; this is abnormal. Note that the normally abnormal appearance of lead aVR, which is unaffected by this left-sided electrode reversal, adds to the subtlety of detection of this entity.

Precordial electrode misconnection and misplacement

If the limb leads are prone to misconnection, then the precordial electrodes are also vulnerable to this error. Precordial electrode misconnection is easy to decipher, however; what is more problematic is precordial electrode misplacement.

Precordial electrode misconnection—usually the inadvertent swapping of two precordial electrodes—results in an interruption of the normal graded transition of R-wave growth and S-wave regression as one scans the precordial leads from right (V1) to left (V6). Moreover, this normal transition is reverted back to in the next electrode that is placed properly [3,5]. When the ECG seems to have a new T-wave change or change in QRS amplitude/ morphology in just one or two precordial leads, it is thus wise to consider precordial electrode reversal. It should be routine practice to survey the R- and S-wave transitions across the precordial leads when first examining the ECG to exclude precordial electrode misconnection.

Similarly, new T-wave changes or changes in the QRS complex may be caused by precordial electrode misplacement—a common problem given that each individual's chest anatomy is unique, making correct anatomic placement a challenge in some cases. When new Q waves, ST segment changes, or T-wave changes are encountered on an ECG being compared with a baseline tracing, one must examine "the company it keeps." For example, when comparing new and old tracings, if a new T-wave inversion occurs in lead V3 with no change in those seen in V4–V6, the amplitude and morphology of the QRS complexes in lead V3 should be compared between the two tracings. If the QRS complexes are dissimilar between the two tracings, it is possible that the precordial electrodes—and here specifically the V3 electrode—were placed differently on the two occasions. Placement of the right precordial electrodes V1 and V2 an interspace too high or too low may result in the appearance or masking, respectively, of an incomplete right bundle branch block pattern [8].

Artifact

Electrocardiographic artifact is a commonly encountered phenomenon and in most cases is recognized easily. Often caused by patient movement (voluntary or involuntary), other sources should be considered, such as 60 cycle-per-second interference from nearby sources of alternating current and electrode and cable problems. Electrode performance is enhanced by connection to dry, non-hairy skin away from bony prominences [9,10].

More challenging and clinically significant is the differentiation of electrocardiographic artifact from real disease, such as dysrhythmia (Fig. 9). Several key features have been advanced that favor pseudodysrhythmia over true dysrhythmia, including (1) absence of symptomatology or hemodynamic variation during the event, (2) normal ventricular complexes appearing among dysrhythmic beats, (3) association with body movement, (4) instability of baseline tracing during and immediately following the alleged dysrhythmia, and (5) synchronous, visible notching consistent with the underlying ventricular rhythm marching through the pseudodysrhythmia [8,11,12].

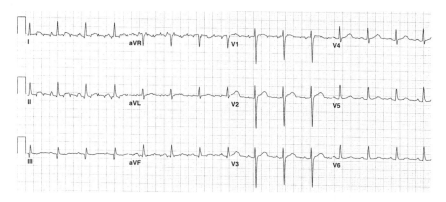

Fig. 9. Patient movement artifact mimicking dysrhythmia. This tracing was recorded on an asymptomatic patient who presented to the ED looking for a psychiatric medication refill. Several leads (I, II, V1, aVF, and aVR) demonstrate what seems to be flutter waves at a rate of 300 bpm. Closer inspection of other leads (III and V3–V6) reveals normal sinus rhythm. The flutter waves were secondary to the patient's parkinsonian tremor, likely resulting from neuroleptic use.

Summary

The ECG can be affected by processes, such as operator error and environmental issues, that are not reflective of yet may mimic underlying disease. As such, the emergency physician should be aware of the manifestations of common limb electrode misconnections, electrode misplacement, and artifact.

References

[1] Surawicz B. Assessing abnormal ECG patterns in the absence of heart disease. Cardiovascular Med 1977;2:629.

[2] Kors JA, van Herpen G. Accurate detection of electrode interchange in the electrocardiogram. Am J Cardiol 2001;88:396.

[3] Surawicz B, Knilans TK. Chou's electrocardiography in clinical practice. 5th edition. Philadelphia: WB Saunders; 2001.

[4] Ho KKL, Ho SK. Use of the sinus P wave in diagnosing electrocardiographic limb lead misplacement not involving the right leg (ground) lead. J Electrocardiol 2001;34:161–71.

[5] Peberdy MA, Ornato JP. Recognition of electrocardiographic lead misplacements. Am J Emerg Med 1993;11:403–5.

[6] Haisty WK, Pahlm O, Edenbrandt L, et al. Recognition of electrocardiographic electrode misplacements involving the ground (right leg) electrode. Am J Cardiol 1993;71:1490–4.

[7] Abdollah H, Milliken JA. Recognition of electrocardiographic left arm/left leg lead reversal. Am J Cardiol 1997;80:1247–9.

[8] Harper RJ, Richards CF. Electrode misplacement and artifact. In: Chan TC, Brady WJ, Harrigan RA, et al, editors. ECG in emergency medicine and acute care. Philadelphia: Elsevier Mosby; 2005. p. 16–21.

[9] Surawica B. Assessing abnormal ECG patterns in the absence of heart disease. Cardiovasc Med 1977;2:629.

[10] Chase C, Brady WJ. Artifactual electrocardiographic change mimicking clinical abnormality on the ECG. Am J Emerg Med 2000;18:312.

[11] Lin SL, Wang SP, Kong CW, et al. Artifact simulating ventricular and atrial arrhythmia. Jpn Heart J 1991;32:847.

[12] Littman L, Monroe MH. Electrocardiographic artifact [letter]. N Engl J Med 2000;342:590.

ELSEVIER
SAUNDERS

EMERGENCY
MEDICINE
CLINICS OF
NORTH AMERICA

Emerg Med Clin N Am 24 (2006) 237–241

Index

Note: Page numbers of article titles are in **boldface** type.

A

Accelerated idioventricular rhythm, 33, 34

Aneurysm, left ventricular, ECG patterns in, 102–103, 104

Aortic dissection, classification of, 137
  description of, 137
  ECG manifestations of, 137–138

Aortic regurgitation, conditions leading to, 125
  ECG findings in, 125

Aortic stenosis, clinical manifestations of, 123–124
  ECG findings in, 125

Atrial fibrillation, 21–23, 24

Atrial flutter, 17–19

Atrial tachycardia, 15–16
  multifocal, 21, 23

Atrioventricular block, 6–9

Atrioventricular conduction blocks, bradydysrhythmias and, **1–9**

B

Beta-adrenergic blocker toxicity, background of, 172–173
  ECG manifestations of, 173
  management of, 173–174

Beta-adrenergic blocking drugs, 172–173

Bifascicular blocks, 45

Bradycardia, 1

Bradycardia-tachycardia syndrome, 5–6

Bradydysrhythmias, 1–6
  and atrioventricular conduction blocks, **1–9**

Brugada syndrome, 43–44, 104
  ECG abnormalities in, 120–121, 122, 123

Bundle branch block(s), acute myocardial infarction and, 49–50
  left, 47, 54, 78, 79, 100, 101
  rate-dependent, 49
  right, 42–44, 46, 79, 99, 100
    differential diagnosis of, 42, 43
  uncomplicated, 99

C

Calcium channel blocker toxicity, background of, 170–171
  ECG manifestations of, 171–172
  management of, 172

Cardiac transplantation, ECG following, 121–123, 124

Cardiomyopathy, hypertrophic, in children, 206

Central nervous system, disease of, ECG changes in, 138–140

Chest pain, ECG in evaluation of, 91

Child(ren), pediatric ECG and, **195–208**

Cholecystitis, ECG findings in, 141

Conduction abnormalities, pediatric ECG and, 202–203

Coronary syndromes, acute, **53–89**
  and ECG ST segment and T wave abnormalities, distinction of, 107–109
  not as cause of ECG ST segment and T abnormalities, **91–111**
  regional issues in, 71–80
  reperfusion therapy in, pathologic Q waves for, 70–71

D

Dextrocardia, ECG manifestations of, 120

Digitalis effect, 105, 106

Changing Your Address?

Make sure your subscription changes too! When you notify us of your new address, you can help make our job easier by including an exact copy of your Clinics label number with your old address (see illustration below.) This number identifies you to our computer system and will speed the processing of your address change. Please be sure this label number accompanies your old address and your corrected address—you can send an old Clinics label with your number on it or just copy it exactly and send it to the address listed below.

We appreciate your help in our attempt to give you continuous coverage. Thank you.

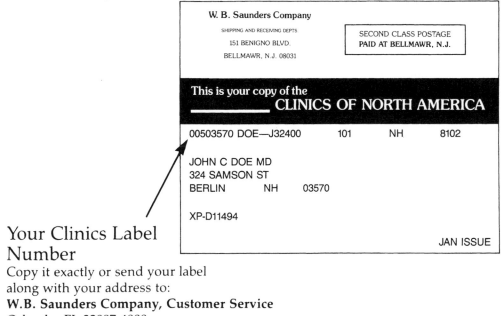

Your Clinics Label Number

Copy it exactly or send your label along with your address to:
W.B. Saunders Company, Customer Service
Orlando, FL 32887-4800
Call Toll Free 1-800-654-2452

Please allow four to six weeks for delivery of new subscriptions and for processing address changes.

United States Postal Service
Statement of Ownership, Management, and Circulation

1. Publication Title	2. Publication Number								3. Filing Date
Emergency Medicine Clinics of North America	0	7	3	3	-	8	6	2	7	9/15/05

4. Issue Frequency	5. Number of Issues Published Annually	6. Annual Subscription Price
Feb, May, Aug, Nov	4	$170.00

7. Complete Mailing Address of Known Office of Publication (Not printer) (Street, city, county, state, and ZIP+4)

Elsevier Inc.
6277 Sea Harbor Drive
Orlando, FL 32887-4800

Contact Person
Gwen C. Campbell
Telephone
215-239-3685

8. Complete Mailing Address of Headquarters or General Business Office of Publisher (Not printer)

Elsevier Inc., 360 Park Avenue South, New York, NY 10010-1710

9. Full Names and Complete Mailing Addresses of Publisher, Editor, and Managing Editor (Do not leave blank)
Publisher (Name and complete mailing address)

Tim Griswold, Elsevier Inc., 1600 John F. Kennedy Blvd., Suite 1800, Philadelphia, PA 19103-2899
Editor (Name and complete mailing address)

Karen Sorensen, Elsevier Inc., 1600 John F. Kennedy Blvd., Suite 1800, Philadelphia, PA 19103-2899
Managing Editor (Name and complete mailing address)

Heather Cullen, Elsevier Inc., 1600 John F. Kennedy Blvd., Suite 1800, Philadelphia, PA 19103-2899

10. Owner (Do not leave blank. If the publication is owned by a corporation, give the name and address of the corporation immediately followed by the names and addresses of all stockholders owning or holding 1 percent or more of the total amount of stock. If not owned by a corporation, give the names and addresses of the individual owners. If owned by a partnership or other unincorporated firm, give its name and address as well as those of each individual owner. If the publication is published by a nonprofit organization, give its name and address.)

Full Name	Complete Mailing Address
Wholly owned subsidiary of	4520 East-West Highway
Reed/Elsevier Inc., US Holdings	Bethesda, MD 20814

11. Known Bondholders, Mortgagees, and Other Security Holders Owning or Holding 1 Percent or More of Total Amount of Bonds, Mortgages, or Other Securities. If none, check box ▶ ☐ None

Full Name	Complete Mailing Address
N/A	

12. Tax Status (For completion by nonprofit organizations authorized to mail at nonprofit rates) (Check one)
The purpose, function, and nonprofit status of this organization and the exempt status for federal income tax purposes:
☐ Has Not Changed During Preceding 12 Months
☐ Has Changed During Preceding 12 Months (Publisher must submit explanation of change with this statement)

(See Instructions on Reverse)

PS Form 3526, October 1999

---

13. Publication Title	14. Issue Date for Circulation Data Below
Emergency Medicine Clinics of North America	August 2005

15.	Extent and Nature of Circulation	Average No. Copies Each Issue During Preceding 12 Months	No. Copies of Single Issue Published Nearest to Filing Date
a.	Total Number of Copies (Net press run)	3225	3000
b. Paid and/or Requested Circulation	(1) Paid/Requested Outside-County Mail Subscriptions Stated on Form 3541. (Include advertiser's proof and exchange copies)	2034	1952
	(2) Paid In-County Subscriptions Stated on Form 3541 (Include advertiser's proof and exchange copies)		
	(3) Sales Through Dealers and Carriers, Street Vendors, Counter Sales, and Other Non-USPS Paid Distribution	365	386
	(4) Other Classes Mailed Through the USPS		
c.	Total Paid and/or Requested Circulation [Sum of 15b. (1), (2), (3), and (4)] ▲	2399	2338
d. Free Distribution by Mail (Samples, complimentary, and other free)	(1) Outside-County as Stated on Form 3541	102	103
	(2) In-County as Stated on Form 3541		
	(3) Other Classes Mailed Through the USPS		
e.	Free Distribution Outside the Mail (Carriers or other means)		
f.	Total Free Distribution (Sum of 15d. and 15e.) ▲	102	103
g.	Total Distribution (Sum of 15c. and 15f.) ▲	2501	2441
h.	Copies not Distributed	724	559
i.	Total (Sum of 15g. and h.) ▲	3225	3000
j.	Percent Paid and/or Requested Circulation (15c. divided by 15g. times 100)	96%	96%

16. Publication of Statement of Ownership
☐ Publication required. Will be printed in the **November 2005** issue of this publication.   ☐ Publication not required

17. Signature and Title of Editor, Publisher, Business Manager, or Owner   Date

(signature) Joan Fanucci – Executive Director of Subscription Services   9/15/05

I certify that all information furnished on this form is true and complete. I understand that anyone who furnishes false or misleading information on this form or who omits material or information requested on the form may be subject to criminal sanctions (including fines and imprisonment) and/or civil sanctions (including civil penalties).

Instructions to Publishers

1. Complete and file one copy of this form with your postmaster annually on or before October 1. Keep a copy of the completed form for your records.
2. In cases where the stockholder or security holder is a trustee, include in items 10 and 11 the name of the person or corporation for whom the trustee is acting. Also include the names and addresses of individuals who are stockholders who own or hold 1 percent or more of the total amount of bonds, mortgages, or other securities of the publishing corporation. In item 11, if none, check the box. Use blank sheets if more space is required.
3. Be sure to furnish all circulation information called for in item 15. Free circulation must be shown in items 15d, e, and f.
4. Item 15h., Copies not Distributed, must include (1) newsstand copies originally stated on Form 3541, and returned to the publisher, (2) estimated returns from news agents, and (3), copies for office use, leftovers, spoiled, and all other copies not distributed.
5. If the publication had Periodicals authorization as a general or requester publication, this Statement of Ownership, Management, and Circulation must be published; it must be printed in any issue in October or, if the publication is not published during October, the first issue printed after October.
6. In item 16, indicate the date of the issue in which this Statement of Ownership will be published.
7. Item 17 must be signed.
Failure to file or publish a statement of ownership may lead to suspension of Periodicals authorization.

PS Form 3526, October 1999 (Reverse)